WHEN MY TIME COMES

WHEN MY TIME COMES

CONVERSATIONS ABOUT WHETHER THOSE WHO ARE DYING SHOULD HAVE THE RIGHT TO DETERMINE WHEN LIFE SHOULD END

DIANE REHM

WHEELER PUBLISHING
A part of Gale, a Cengage Company

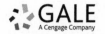

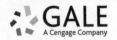

Copyright © 2020 by Diane Rehm.
Wheeler Publishing, a part of Gale, a Cengage Company.

ALL RIGHTS RESERVED
Wheeler Publishing Large Print Hardcover.
The text of this Large Print edition is unabridged.
Other aspects of the book may vary from the original edition.
Set in 16 pt. Plantin.

**LIBRARY OF CONGRESS CIP DATA ON FILE.
CATALOGUING IN PUBLICATION FOR THIS BOOK
IS AVAILABLE FROM THE LIBRARY OF CONGRESS**

ISBN-13: 978-1-4328-8109-2 (hardcover alk. paper)

Published in 2021 by arrangement with Alfred A. Knopf, an imprint of The Knopf Doubleday Publishing Group, a division of Penguin Random House LLC

Printed in Mexico
Print Number: 01   Print Year: 2020

This book is dedicated, first,
to the memory of my late husband,
John Rehm.
Our long marriage, and his death,
have shaped my life;
to my husband of two years,
John Hagedorn,
who has brought new joy into my life;
finally, to my beloved children,
David and Jennifer Rehm,
and their families

CONTENTS

7

FOREWORD
JOHN GRISHAM

I believe it's wrong to sustain a life beyond the point when it should not be sustained, when it should be terminated. We all are aware of cases of people being kept alive by modern medicine long past the time when they should be allowed to die. I think that it becomes immoral if a person is brain dead, clinically dead, and is being kept alive by machines. This is something that my wife and I have always felt strongly about.

She and I have been fortunate. We haven't had a relative or close friend go through a prolonged and drawn-out death that should not have been allowed. After open and honest discussions with our parents years ago, we encouraged them to execute living wills and get these things on file so that they would not be sustained against their wishes by modern medicine. They had witnessed the other — the bad — side of things, and knew how awful it can be. I'm sure it's hard

11

for some families to have such discussions, but our parents — very alive, very healthy at the time — were determined to avoid being kept alive when they wanted to die.

As for my wife and me, we've made certain that our schoolteacher daughter and lawyer son are very clear about how we feel about prolonging life when it shouldn't be prolonged, and our son has copies of our living wills and advance directives in his office. This is something we've talked about with the kids over a long period of time, and since we all feel the same way, that's been easy for us to do. And we've encouraged *them* to do the right paperwork, too — living wills — and get those on file, because calamitous things can strike one at any age. They don't just happen to old people. Young people, too, can get injured, have strokes or heart attacks or even worse diseases, and can linger hopelessly and painfully for a long, long time.

I've heard the argument that right to die laws could be used to pressure old or disabled people to die, but I've never been exposed to a case like that. I appreciate the argument, and can imagine that it could happen in a very small percentage of cases, but for me the benefits of allowing a person to choose far outweighs the risk. As for the idea that someone who stood to inherit from a sick person could force that individual to deploy the right to die laws, I think that there are enough safeguards — other family members, health-care professionals — in place to prevent abuse.

As for me, although I've been lucky enough not to have witnessed anything close to a patient who was suffering terribly and just wanted to end it all, that's kind of my fear — to find myself in a situation where I or a loved one is in a great deal of pain and suffering with no hope of recovery. That's why my wife and I have directed our health-care professionals to not resuscitate and to terminate all treatment in the event that we become terminally ill with no reasonable chance of recovery.

I have a very close friend who's a neurosurgeon, and I know from him the high price doctors pay for dealing so much with death. We drink a bottle of wine together, and he talks about facing so much death and so much suffering, and how doctors and nurses in these situations know what to do. Not that he comes out with details, but I can infer that they just know how to manipulate the medications to bring about a peaceful end to someone who is suffering and never going to recover. To me, that's a "good death." I suppose I'm a coward. Just crank up the morphine and put me to sleep!

When I was a young lawyer, I had a case where a ten-year-old boy was burned over 95 percent of his body, basically from his eyes and nose all the way down, and they flew him to this specialty hospital where they treated him for a year. They saved his life . . . and for the rest of his life he resented what they had done to him. He was disfigured, he was miserable — it was horrible. I tell my wife that if I get burned terribly and am going to be scarred and disfigured, I don't want to be saved, okay? It's over.

My number one fear, though, is a stroke that leaves me with pretty serious brain damage and unable to do a lot of things, yet still able to live pain-free and to function at some level. But rehab often works for stroke victims — sometimes it's miraculous. So I wouldn't be so quick to pull the plug with a stroke as I would be for people with terminal cancer or Parkinson's or Alzheimer's disease. Alzheimer's gets to me, because you have these people who are physically gone. People who have been lying there for years and are basically brain dead, physically dead, dead, dead. But they're breathing without machines. Their families go through this horrific end of life trying to love and care for someone who's not there. It's also a huge financial burden on our health system.

I'm fortunate because I have my friend the neurosurgeon as a resource. I don't care what my health problem may be, this guy is going to tell me the truth. (I'm sixty-three; he's about ten years older.) He's told me so many stories over the years. For instance, one about a patient with grade-four glioblastomas. He and his doctors have these discussions saying, "You have about a year to live. If you have some surgery or radiation, all the different procedures, you can have about a year. Or you can do nothing, go home, stay comfortable, and you'll have about six months." You'd be surprised how often the advice is "Don't do anything. Don't do surgery because it'll mess you up physically and it's not going to prolong anything but the agony. Yes, miracles happen, we see that all the time. Even so, there's a 95 percent likelihood that you're not going to live more than two years, or something like that." The patient then knows the score and can make his or her decision.

My mother had cancer for the last seven years of her life. It finally got her when she was eighty. Most of those years were good years, and along the way her doctors always leveled with us. She died at home. I was holding one hand, my dad was holding the other. My two sisters and my mom's sister were there — they'd spent the afternoon together — and then she decided it was time to go because it was time to go. So we spent a couple of hours with her in her bed, and then she went as peacefully as could be. I have two brothers, two sisters, and we all had input into Mom's care. Everyone said, "Do not let her suffer. She's not going to get up and start walking again, she's not going to recover" — we all knew that. I think my sister, who's a nurse, made sure that Mom was never uncomfortable — she was on morphine — and she just went to sleep, and her breathing got more and more labored, slower and slower, and she finally took her last breath. And we were all there. I think of it as a good death.

We were raised very devout believers in God, believers in Christ, very devout Southern Baptists — that's the faith we had. We knew we'd be together in the afterlife. That's why I don't fear death. I know that many religious people believe that right to die laws go against the will of God — that God should be the only decider. To me, the issue depends on *how* you decide. If you are young and healthy and full of promise but have mental issues or depression, and you decide to take your own life, I'm not sure that God would approve. Or that it would be a rational move for you to make. Suicide can be the ultimate act of selfishness because of what it leaves behind, especially if it's by a young person.

What I'm talking about is people who are terminally ill and who are not going to recover — people in pain, facing death; that's a totally different situation, because death is already there. Alzheimer's patients can live for three or four years before they finally conk out, but they're practically dead. Death has arrived. Modern medicine may postpone it . . . that's what I question. If you're stricken with a horrible cancer, that's your fate. I'm not going to say God did it to you. That's your fate. And you're going to die. Not sure when, where, or how, but you're going to go through a process in which your body deteriorates, the cancer takes over, there's going to be a hospital bed with tubes and meds and all that. You are at the end. And you should be able to decide when you're ready to go.

Even if the doctors can keep you comfortable for a little longer, it should be the decision of the patient, assuming that the patient facing a terminal situation is in command of his or her mental faculties. The decision does not belong to the doctor. It belongs to the patient. It's the right to die, and we should all have that right.

PREFACE

Death was part of my life at an early age.

It's December 1955. My beautiful mother lies in a bed at Georgetown University Hospital, crying, moaning, suffering, begging for God to take her. For perhaps the sixth time, she has been drained of several quarts of fluid. Before each procedure, her stomach becomes severely distended, making her appear to be nine months pregnant. I am alone as I watch her, feeling totally helpless, crying as I stroke her feet, unable to ease her pain, hating her suffering, hating that she has to continue living. She is forty-nine years old. I am nineteen. We are told she is suffering from cirrhosis of the liver, a disease ordinarily attributed to alcoholism. My mother is not an alcoholic. She and my father share a shot glass of whiskey on Christmas and New Year's Eve. The doctors are skeptical of her denials, but finally come to believe her. Had they asked me, I could have vouched for my mother's nondrinking habits. I knew she had suffered from malaria in her teenage years, when she lived in Alexandria, Egypt. Whether that disease could have affected her liver to such an extent forty years later, I cannot know. She lay in that hospital bed for weeks, her beautiful unwrinkled skin and eyes yellowed with jaundice, the fluid continually mounting, swelling her belly again and again.

December 31, 1955. My husband and I have just moved into our new apartment, several blocks from my parents' home. We have no telephone. We are planning to go to a New Year's Eve celebration given by our church group, but first we visit my mother at the hospital.

When we arrive at ten p.m., she lies sleeping, with the rails up on each side of her bed. I don't want to wake her, so we silently tiptoe out of the room.

We run into her doctor, who asks whether we've seen her. "We did go in," I say, "but she is asleep and I don't want to wake her." The doctor tells us to go back, to wake her, to be sure she knows I am there. I'm hesitant, but he urges me to return to her room. I do, but she hardly acknowledges me when I wake her. I feel terrible. I don't want to go to a New Year's Eve party, but we do. The doctor knew what he did not tell us: my mother would barely live through the night.

New Year's Day 1956. A loud knocking at our apartment door. It's my husband's brother. He says we must come quickly to the hospital. We race there, speeding, hoping for police to catch us and help us get to Georgetown. I run ahead of my husband and brother-in-law through the parking lot, into the hospital, and to her room. My father, sister, and aunts are there, all weeping. She is still in her bed. But it's too late. She died twenty minutes before we arrive.

My mother begged to die. There was no hope of recovery. There was nothing more they could do to ease her pain or to keep her comfortable. She died suffering.

As a child of six, and for many years thereafter, I can recall saying to my mother, "I want to die before you do. I don't want to live without you." Deep in my heart, I'd known she wasn't well, and I feared being left behind. To then have had to watch her suffer for so long became the beginning of my passionate belief in the right to die.

It began while watching my mother in her agony, feeling so angry that doctors could do nothing to help ease her way into the inevitable. I kept wondering why she had to suffer, why she could not simply be put out

21

of her misery, when there was no cure in sight.

Of course, back in 1955, there were no liver transplants being performed, and no "right to die" laws in place anywhere in the country. It was not until 1998 that Oregon became the first state in the country to adopt such a law. The state of Washington followed in 2009, Montana by a court case in 2009, Vermont in 2013, California in 2015, Colorado in 2016, the District of Columbia in 2017, Hawaii in 2018, and New Jersey and Maine in 2019. Just nine states, plus the District of Columbia, where individuals are permitted to choose when to cease their suffering through the use of medical aid in dying. Now numerous state legislatures are in fierce debate among those who believe, as I do, that each of us has the right to choose when our suffering should end, and those who argue, on religious or moral or ethical grounds, that no human being has the right to hasten an individual's death. The opponents define the right to die as suicide. Other countries, such as Switzerland and the Netherlands, have long had laws allowing doctors to respond to requests of individuals to end their lives, some because of physical illness, others due to severe emotional distress.

For the past two years, I have interviewed many people: patients with terminal illnesses, doctors, nurses, ethicists, and those left behind. They told stories of their journeys through end-of-life preparation, shared their perspectives, and spoke honestly of their beliefs, hopes, and fears. Most will appear in the television documentary *When My Time Comes,* a companion to this book.

Both the book and the film are meant to shed light on the reality of medical aid in dying, the process, who is eligible, what it means for those people who have been approved, the feelings of physicians involved, as well as the thoughts of those left behind.

Those of us who have worked together on the documentary have one goal in mind: to urge a discussion of death, a topic so many fear to mention. This is true in too many families, where the subject of death is never brought up until it is too late, when the reality of a loved one's illness leaves children or siblings with no understanding of what the individual might want. Legal documents indicating "Do not resuscitate" or "Use no artificial means to sustain life" are not enough.

What is required is talk — real, honest-to-goodness talk, not only with family, but also with doctors, ministers, and friends. What do you want when you are near the end of life? Do you wish to die in a hospital after being kept alive by machines and ventilators, with every last medical option being applied to your body, or do you wish to die at home, in your own bed, surrounded by family, and comforted by a caring physician who has provided you with the medication to end your suffering when you decide you've had enough? Those are the conversations I pray this book and the documentary will spur. When those talks reach state legislatures, when the men and women who make such decisions are persuaded of the legitimacy of the individual's right to determine the time for life to end, we will be more at ease in the belief that death is an integral part of life.

BARBARA COOMBS LEE
PRESIDENT, COMPASSION & CHOICES

Barbara Coombs Lee began her medical career as a candy striper at St. Joseph Hospital in Joliet, Illinois. As she writes in her book, *Finish Strong: Putting Your Priorities First at Life's End,* she's been working in health care for almost fifty-five years, specializing in intensive care and emergency rooms, caring for very ill patients, helping them stay alive. However, she came to believe in an individual's right to finish life on his or her own terms. She remembers the day: May 19, 1994, the day Jacqueline Kennedy Onassis died of non-Hodgkin's lymphoma.

She writes: "Her son, John F. Kennedy, Jr., emerged from her apartment that morning and comforted the crowd that stood grieving on Fifth Avenue. He said, 'My mother died surrounded by her friends and her family and her books. She did it in her own way and on her own terms. And we all

25

feel lucky for that.' "

Barbara said that moment motivated her to find a way to avert the suffering that so many undergo at the end of life. She became a public advocate, gaining admission to the Oregon State Bar, and ultimately joining the staff of the Oregon Senate Healthcare and Bioethics Committee. In 1994, the year of her conversion, she became one of the three chief petitioners who filed the Oregon Death with Dignity Act as a citizens' initiative. She writes, "I spent the next fourteen years defending the resulting Death with Dignity law from efforts to undo it in every governmental arena — legislative, executive and judicial."

Oregon's law had been embattled until 2006, when the U.S. Supreme Court finally ruled that states have the authority to adopt medical aid in dying as part of the legitimate practice of medicine.

On February 12, 2019, I interviewed Barbara for my podcast, *On My Mind.*

I began by asking her about the lessons she had learned from caring for people who had not died well, who had had unwanted treatments and been kept alive against their wishes.

"The technology that medicine wields, and of which we are so proud, is not necessarily in an individual's best interest. Only individuals can review their lives, their beliefs, their values, and decide what is best for them. It took many more years and many more bedside experiences in intensive care units, emergency rooms, nursing homes, et cetera, before I had what you might call a broader understanding of people's end-of-life journey. I learned that it might be different for each of us. It's as though medicine has gotten ahead of human desire. There are so many ways to keep us alive, and yet the incredibly sophisticated means of keeping people alive don't always take into account what people themselves want."

Barbara calls dying in America a "terrible mess." She says, "We torture people with treatments that are futile and enormously burdensome, robbing them of the precious quality of their remaining days, robbing them of the time they would otherwise want to devote to the priorities of their lives, the legacy of memories they would like to leave their loved ones. We concentrate on extending the absolute duration of life irrespective of how dismal and degraded and burdensome the quality of that life might be. Something like 30 to 40 percent of people have an ICU admission in the last thirty days of life. Nine out of ten people with dementia — profound dementia — have some sort of invasive procedure. In the last month of life, we are replacing humanity with technology."

DIANE: Tell the story of Maria, an eighty-two-year-old who has do not resuscitate, or DNR, orders. What happened to her?

BARBARA: She had her advance directive. She made sure everyone had the directive and knew she did not want to have any resuscitation efforts applied when she was admitted to the hospital emergency room for some abdominal pain. She had done what we're supposed to do, and she did it in spades. She wanted to make sure that everyone in the hospital knew about her request, and that if some calamity happened during her hospitalization, she would not have to undergo resuscitation efforts. And then, one night, very peacefully, her heart stopped and her advance directive was just ignored. She was given CPR entirely against the likelihood that she would be revived. She *was* revived and taken to the ICU, and her son and grandson were told what had happened to her. And they visited her in the ICU, and she was devastated. She was alert. She was angry. She couldn't speak because there were tubes in her mouth and down her throat. But she knew she had been violated.

D: But how could this happen? If she went into the hospital with an advance directive, why was it ignored? How frequently does that happen?

B: The sad truth, Diane, is that advance directives are often ignored, particularly in situations like this, when a sudden catastrophe occurs. Advance directives on their face apply in two circumstances. If a person is terminally ill or permanently unconscious, that's when medical providers are told to honor the wishes of the patient. Well, physicians are loath to say that someone is "terminally ill" or "permanently unconscious." I would venture to say that even if Maria's physicians were aware there was an advance directive and a desire to refuse CPR, they would have ignored it anyway, because in their minds, she's not terminally ill. They think they're going to bring her back! She's just having a little spell, and they can bring her around. In legal terms, the conditions of terminal illness or permanent unconsciousness in her advance directive have not been met.

D: That makes me wonder whether if something were to happen to me — if I'm having a heart attack or a stroke — I would really want to go to a hospital.

B: There's a balance. If I see someone drop down on the sidewalk in front of me and her heart has stopped, I wouldn't consult her advance directive either. I'd give her a good thump and see if I can restart her heart. But in very short order, someone needs to inquire what the person's desires are. Would he or she want a vigorous resuscitation effort? And for how long? The atrocity that was committed on Maria was not that she got one shock, but that she was held captive in the ICU and they refused to take her off these machines and take out the tubes, even when she communicated by hand squeezes. They did not honor her specific instruction.

D: Had Maria been in a religiously affiliated hospital?

B: No. I think it's more indicative of the prevailing mentality and the desire of the medical community to not give up too soon. The determination to bring her back. Compare Maria's story with Lorraine Bayless, the woman who had the "good fortune" to die on the cafeteria floor of her independent living facility. She was not subjected to CPR because it was not the facility's policy, but someone called 911. And once 911 was involved, all the death aversion in our society and our nation swept full force into the cafeteria. The 911 operator just would not let go. I think the woman was about eighty-five, and she'd had a sudden massive stroke. She was very close to death. And the people around her wanted someone to breathe into her mouth or get paddles.

D: As I recall from your book, the care facility in which the woman resided was prohibited from doing anything to actively try to resuscitate. Articles then appeared in *The New York Times* and elsewhere calling the institution cruel because it did not lift a finger to resuscitate.

B: Right. You know, I wish I could pull up some of those news clips where very young journalists on the evening news were opining that this woman had been terribly abused, that in spite of her advanced age she would've been likely to bounce back from a total collapse of her cerebral vascular and cardiovascular systems and go on to lead a high-quality life for many years, and that the institution depriving her of this opportunity was criminal.

Her daughters came to the situation with much more common sense and an intimate knowledge of their mother and her desires. They said, "We are not litigious people. Moreover, our mom knew what she wanted. She wanted to be in an institution where she could die peacefully. And so we won't be suing anyone for granting her wish."

D: What exactly are you advising people to do, so that they can "finish strong"?

B: Finish in a way that aligns with your priorities. Make sure it is a fitting closure to your values and beliefs. My book is really not a book about dying. It's a book about living. It's a book about living fully and not being abducted onto a conveyor belt of medical technology that leads to a robbing of your priorities, and a displacement of the things that you value most at the end of life. Live your last precious months or weeks, or even years, according to the things that give you the most joy.

D: I believe that one of the critical elements of "finishing strong" is having a conversation with children, parents, loved ones, and friends as to exactly what you want. There are so many people reluctant to raise the subject. It's the last taboo. We don't talk about death. I remember speaking in a church in Massachusetts. There were about three or four hundred people in the congregation, and I began by saying, "Please raise your hand if you plan not to die." And of course there was great giggling in the audience, but it was an uncomfortable giggling. People just don't want to raise the subject. How do we get past that?

B: I would say it's not just one conversation but many conversations, an ongoing dialogue. That includes recording your values and priorities in a video or on your iPhone or something, so that people will remember. It's hard to have a conversation about what I want because there are so many variables, depending on what situation I find myself in.

But what will guide people is what I cherish. I think the most important thing we can tell our loved ones is "If you are asked to make decisions when I cannot, know this above all: My values. Know what I hold to be most sacred in my life that I would never want to give up. And if I cannot reclaim that, if the likelihood of my reclaiming that in the future is very low, then act accordingly." Now there's a lot of emphasis on when these decisions are made for me by someone else. But the truth of the matter is that most decisions that get us in trouble, that put us on the conveyor belt of futile and burdensome care, that rob us of the quality of our life, we make ourselves when we are conscious and capable of making health-care decisions. But all too often, we just don't have enough information to make those decisions in a smart way. We don't understand what we're getting into, and we don't understand that we can hop off the conveyor belt at some time in the future. So we must learn to ask questions.

We must learn to ask, when any test

or treatment is proposed, how efficacious it is, how many people in my situation are cured by this treatment, how many have had their lives extended by this treatment. *Zero to 2 percent.* Extended by how much? *Well, by three to four weeks.* At what cost? What are the burdens of this treatment? How much time does it take? How will I feel afterward? Will I be able to do the things I enjoy? We make those decisions, we sign the consent form and say, "Yes, sign me up to do this treatment." But we don't realize that it may be futile and it may be robbing us of our quality of life and our precious time.

D: Should right to die laws apply to people with Alzheimer's disease, or is that a step too far?

B: Medical aid in dying is hard to apply to people with Alzheimer's, because it's hard to imagine delivering a life-ending medication to people who don't know that they're taking it, or aren't physically capable of taking it. I don't think that the American people are likely to adopt a policy like that in the near future. But I would say this: The fact that medical aid in dying does not apply to people with dementia or Alzheimer's is not the real problem. The real problem is all the things we currently do to delay the natural process of dying.

My book speaks honestly about how one might make a plan to escape dementia — not endure and fail to cope with dementia but escape it. If a threshold of unacceptable deterioration is approaching, there are so many ways to invite an intended death without resorting to some lethal medication that is delivered by a third party. Most people with advanced dementia have some kind of invasive procedure to keep them alive, in most cases not something they would have chosen. We're not allowing nature to take its course. If there is an infection, we treat it. If there is pneumonia, we treat it. If people aren't drinking and they're dehydrated, we start IVs and we rehydrate them. We might spend a year sustaining the bodily functions that would normally decline and stop altogether if we allowed the disease to take its natural course. I say there's no shame, there's no guilt in having and articulating an intention to die. If I am not actually living, but only existing, I want my loved ones to act on that intention, and if I am still capable, I will act on that intention, if I see this threshold approaching.

D: I spoke clearly to my grandson while he recorded me on a cell phone, to let him and others know my wish if I begin to feel the effects and recognize the effects of dementia coming on. Thus I have it on record for family that I do not wish to survive the end stages of dementia. It's so important, as you say, to think about what happens down the line; not just for today, but as time goes on.

B: Good for you, Diane. That's brilliant. We're working right now on a tool at Compassion & Choices called the Dementia Decoder that will help people anticipate what may be in store for them. Help people pinpoint the threshold they do not wish to cross and help make it very clear to others around them that yes, they want this information, they want to know when that threshold is approaching and then want to be able to implement steps so that the progression doesn't continue beyond that threshold. It takes a clear-eyed determination, and I know you have it. It takes a loving family. And it takes some thought and some articulation so that people are armed with the knowledge they need and the tools to act on it when that threshold approaches.

LORI WALLACE-PUSHINAITIS
TERMINAL CANCER PATIENT
&
DR. CATHERINE SONQUIST FOREST
CLINICAL ASSOCIATE PROFESSOR OF MEDICINE, UNIVERSITY OF CALIFORNIA, SAN FRANCISCO, NATIVIDAD MEDICAL CENTER, LORI'S END-OF-LIFE CARE DOCTOR

When I first walk into Lori Wallace-Pushinaitis's apartment in San Jose, I realize the entire living room is so small that the video-recording equipment fills most of the space. She and Dr. Forest are seated close together on a wooden bench, chatting easily with each other, as though they are very dear friends. Lori's head is wrapped in a pale blue scarf, I assume because she has lost all her hair. She is very pale, without eyebrows or eyelashes. There are small pieces of folk art decorating the wall, and behind Lori and Dr. Forest are glass doors leading to an area where Lori has been potting plants for her patio.

Lori Wallace was born and raised in San Jose, California. She gave birth to her first child at age nineteen, just as she began college, and put herself through college as a welfare mother, working two or three jobs at a time. She became an environmental professional, describing herself as "one of those people . . . already eating organic and being this hippie girl that's super-healthy. But I still got breast cancer when I was thirty-nine. I was working for the city of San Jose, managing residential-waste collection and processing contracts. I've had cancer for a little over seven years."

I ask Lori about the kind of treatment she has received.

"My breast cancer has metastasized, which means it's gone outside the breast and there is no cure. All treatment is palliative, to extend life and relieve the pain of cancer. It's a miracle that I'm still alive. I'm forty-six and have had cancer for seven years. It's been metastatic for a little over four years. I have the BRCA2 gene, which I inherited from my mother's side of the family — so many of my family members died of breast cancer that I knew there was a good chance I would get it. I did all the preventive things I could. I started eating organic, I took good care of myself, but having done those appropriate things, I still developed breast cancer."

Dr. Forest met Lori at Stanford Health Care. Dr. Forest was one of the founders of Stanford's program for handling requests for exercising the End of Life Option Act in California, which legalized medical aid in dying and went into effect in June 2016. She has been speaking to other doctors around the country about medical aid in dying.

When Lori discovered she was possibly within the six-month window of terminal, she made the request for medical aid in dying. When the two women met, Dr. Forest reassured Lori that she would stay with her throughout the process, and would continue to evaluate her. Although Lori has already outlived that six-month window required to apply for medical aid in dying, Dr. Forest told Lori she could make the decision to ask for the medication at any time, or to revoke that decision at any time.

Dr. Forest understands that having that option is a comfort for Lori. Together the two have spoken with Lori's family, who are also aware that Lori has that option and can revoke it at any time. Like Lori, many people outlive their first six-month diagnosis, so, said Dr. Forest, "We just extend that time line and stay connected and evaluate

41

for as long as she remains competent and able to take the medication herself."

DIANE: That must give you some re-assurance.

LORI: Well, I know that I'm dying. I've known that for four years. And one of the scariest things about that is, you have no control, right? No one can fix it, no one can make it better. All my life I've been a control freak. But it doesn't work with cancer. However, now I can control how I die. If I could choose when to die, it would be when I'm ninety. But that's not an option. I have very distinct memories of my great-grandmother dying of Alzheimer's, and by the time I was six, I knew I did not want to die like that. Watching what happened to my great-grandmother terrified me of the possibility of losing my personality and myself. Death has been part of my whole life. My aunt died horribly of breast cancer, and that's not what I want.

D: Are you in pain?

L: Absolutely, ever since I first felt my lump and self-diagnosed. I woke up in the middle of the night, and I rolled over and had this stabbing pain in my chest, and I thought it was one of my little boy's toys. So I brushed it away and the pain was still there. I thought, Well, that's not right. So I ended up having an incisional biopsy, just taking the whole lump out, because it hurt.

I don't want to die. I'm just forced to deal with dying, even though I prefer to try to spend as much of my time as I can just living. When you first find out you're terminal, death hangs over you, like it's this overwhelming darkness. It shuts out the sunlight. But death can't overshadow you forever, right?

D: Tell me about the first time you met Dr. Forest.

L: I already knew that I wanted to take advantage of the End of Life Option Act. I've always thought there should be options for people at the end. So the minute I found out that the legislation was being considered, I told my oncologist: I want you to put in your notes that I want this option, and she's like, It's not even passed yet. And I say, I don't care. I want there to be as long a history in my medical records as possible, so that there's no way anyone can

43

question my decision or say that some-one was pressuring me. If things start going really bad, I don't want to suffer weeks or months of misery.

Dr. Forest tells me that Lori does not have the necessary drugs now, but the prescription could be ready within forty-eight hours. That's the number one thing people are concerned about, she says, the amount of lag time when you need the drugs. She says Lori is fierce around pain, but it's not for her physician to determine the extent of her suffering — that Lori is the one to make the judgment.

I asked Dr. Forest why she had become supportive of medical aid in dying.

DR. FOREST: I trained in San Francisco at the height of the AIDS era. I've been a family medicine doctor more than twenty-five years now, and I've had many patients ask me for this, for aid in dying. Palliative care, hospice care — there's a whole group of options. But in my experience, there's a subgroup of people for whom nothing that we can do helps with their suffering at the end of life — nothing. And medical aid in dying does. There's been this sort of quiet ability in the medical profession to employ medical treatments that hasten death. We can take people off life support. That hastens death. People can stop eating and drinking, and that hastens death. It's not medical treatments.

I witnessed my own grandmother's death. She was a physician, the first female chief of staff of a hospital in the U.S. And she ended up, against her will, on life support. It was a difficult time for my family. She never would have made that choice — she would have chosen aid in dying. So my grandmother, my grandfather, my mother, and I said at that time that we would fight for it to become legal. My grandmother died during my first year of medical school, but we'd already had conversations about what our choices would be at the end of life. And she was very much in support of patient autonomy. Yet she ended up in a situation that she would never have chosen.

D: Why did the doctors make that decision without the family being present?

DR. F: She was brought into the hospital in an emergency situation. If she were here today, she would very much support medical aid in dying, as would my grandfather, also a physician.

The very day I interviewed Lori and Dr. Forest, the California law was challenged and put on hold indefinitely. I asked Dr. Forest what she would do while the hold was in place.

DR. F: As a licensed physician in the state of California I practice within the confines of what's legal. And if aid in dying becomes illegal again, I'll be back in the same situation: I will not write prescriptions.

D: But you said earlier than many deaths do take place "under the table" when suffering is present?

DR. F: Yes. But very quietly and clandestinely. For instance, in hospice I was trained to go ahead and turn up the medication for my AIDS patients to ease suffering, knowing that it would hasten death. I think the statistic is that more or less one-third of practicing physicians would say that they've seen or done that themselves.

D: I hope — for Lori's sake, for my own sake, and for everyone's sake — that the law is not overturned. I worry about that very vocal minority who would like to see it overturned. Dr. Forest, do you think that's a possibility?

DR. F: I think you're right to be worried, because the tactics that are used in opposition to privacy and patient autonomy are formidable elements of our society. Given the last year and a half in California and twenty years in Oregon, and that this is very compassionate medical care for the people for whom it's appropriate, it would be a tragedy to go back to when they did not have control over their own suffering at the very end of their lives.

D: Lori, would you use the medication if you had it?

L: I don't know. I don't know how things are going to look when I'm dying. I would love to fall asleep and then die in my sleep, but if it gets to the point where I have no quality of life and cannot have my pain treated, I'm going to want to do something about that. I'm incredibly stubborn, and I don't take no for an answer very well. I would find a way to make it happen. You know, before this law in California passed, I used to think, Well, what part of Highway 1 has a cliff that you can just drive off, because I don't want a prolonged death. Not only for me, but also for my children. I have a twelve-year-old and he does not need to see his mother in misery, screaming and crying and not myself, in a situation where all he's going to get is trauma and misery. That's not okay.

D: How does your husband feel about your decision?

L: He supports me 100 percent.

When Lori underwent breast-removal surgery, she was told she had no lymph node involvement and only about a 10 percent chance of recurrence. She then discovered she had the BRCA2 gene, and decided to do a prophylactic bilateral mastectomy. At that point she was very hopeful about living to a ripe old age. But fourteen months later she discovered that her cancer was metastatic.

L: My biggest concern when I found out that I was metastatic was that there's no way to control my pain, because I can't take opiates — they make me crazy. And I don't want to be that person.

D: Dr. Forest, what, as a physician, would you say to the patient or family when there is nothing more that can be done? Do you actually tell a patient: *You are terminal?*

DR. F: The short answer is yes. Having these kinds of conversations about prognosis is crucial. I don't know how long someone is going to live, but statistics are helpful in that they help someone plan for kind of the worst-case scenario. I ask questions about what a patient wants to do, what kinds of goals she might have, would treatment keep you from being with your kids. Developing a prognosis is not an exact science, but giving people a sense of how much time they have is liberating. They can live the life that they have.

D: Describe the prescription terminally ill people receive, if they have met all the criteria for medical aid in dying.

DR. F: The prescription itself, of a controlled substance, is a compounded mixture of drugs we can easily get. Once I write that prescription, it's out of my hands in terms of what someone does with it. It's a faith, it's a trust, it's a culture of honesty that the patient will respect and protect the medication and use it as directed. The prescription is valid for one month. The medication is not in capsule or tablet form. It's in a compounded liquid and has been described as tasting absolutely vile.

I wondered whether this is because the medical profession wants to make sure you really want to take it and are willing to ingest this god-awful-tasting stuff.

Dr. Forest responded that she didn't believe the taste was calculated to be disagreeable, and added that small user groups are sharing information about how to remove that acidic, biting, bitter taste.

I asked Lori how she felt, knowing about the awful taste of the end-of-life medication.

L: I have endured more than most humans can imagine, so in my world, I don't even care. Death is going to be a hard pill to swallow in that I don't want to die anyway.

D: Dr. Forest, could you describe end-of-life suffering?

DR. F: You can't be in practice for decades as a family physician and not be present both at the beginning and at the end of life. Most people have a vision that they'll just comfortably slip away. Before 1950, most people died suddenly. The age people lived to was around sixty or seventy, and people would die of a stroke or heart attack or an accident or infection. What's happened now, in my experience, is that people die slowly. They die of cancer, heart disease, strokes, and infections, but after extended periods of time. As a consequence the suffering is different for different people. Sometimes they have pain we just cannot palliate. Or they have the best care in the world and they still experience physical pain. It might be psychological pain or spiritual pain, very difficult to treat medically. For some, the loss of dignity and autonomy is more than they can bear. So it's a different kind of suffering. To bear witness to that is excruciating for the family, and certainly for the person experiencing it. I've seen people unable to catch their breath. Not being able to address that suffering, whatever it is, is just heartbreaking for a physician.

I believe the best thing we can do is to support people who are willing to embrace an expansion of medical practice to include this kind of treatment of suffering. Tell the stories of suffering that don't fit into the medical model, tell stories of how the option itself gives you a sense of relief, like you could do something, you could have autonomy at the end of your life. Telling those stories is crucial.

Letting legislators know you are in support of aid in dying is not minor. These laws get passed because legislators know their constituents want them. If we as physicians don't speak out, then legislators don't know they can actually push back against the very vocal minority. It's not until you're faced with death yourself, either as a patient or as someone personally involved with one that you become aware of the limitations or barriers.

We are working on a national curriculum for medical schools. One out of five Americans now lives in a state where medical aid in dying is legal. People need to know about it, whether they're going to deploy it or not. The training doesn't exist in very many places yet, but I think it's being raised as an issue.

Lori Wallace-Pushinaitis died on October 20, 2018. At the end she decided to have hospice in the last days and passed away just as she had hoped to — surrounded by loved ones — without the use of medical aid in dying.

CHRISTINA PUCHALSKI

BOARD-CERTIFIED PALLIATIVE-CARE PHYSICIAN, GERIATRICIAN, AND INTERNIST, GEORGE WASHINGTON UNIVERSITY SCHOOL OF MEDICINE

Dr. Christina Puchalski is the daughter of Polish immigrants, the first member of the family born in the United States. Her parents witnessed the devastation of World War II in Poland. Her mother escaped to England with her son and her first husband, who was later killed. Dr. Puchalski's father was in the underground army, part of the Resistance, instrumental in helping Jewish people get out safely. Her parents met in England after her mother became widowed. Her parents and her brother moved to California, where Dr. Puchalski was born and raised. She has beautiful red hair, very fair skin, and a wonderful smile. She says her parents instilled in her important values about honoring people and respecting everybody, regardless of age or illness or color or race.

DIANE: Dr. Puchalski, tell me about the

work you do now.

DR. PUCHALSKI: When I became a physician, I was struck by the lack of attention to spiritual issues, broadly defined. Not just religious, but spiritual issues, meaning purpose, what people value most in clinical care. I started a course at George Washington University on spirituality and health. Since then, I've worked on research, on developing guidelines for how to address spiritual issues with patients, particularly in palliative care.

D: You were raised Roman Catholic?

DR. P: Yes. I was raised that way, but my parents also valued the importance of beliefs in general. My dad, in particular, was very interested in different spiritual practices. We explored lots of different faiths, and that interest has continued throughout my life.

D: Your father is now ninety-eight years old?

DR. P: Yes. It's absolutely amazing. He's in a wheelchair — he's had a lot of health issues in the last five years, and I believe he is nearing the end of his life. I can see changes in him now: he's a little more contemplative and quieter. At the same time, he has amazing capacity to enjoy. Even last night, as I sat with him on the edge of the bed and he started coughing, the doctor in me was thinking, Is this going to progress to pneumonia and should I call hospice now? He, on the other hand, was fully enjoying the moment. His health aide was on the other side of the bed, and they were sort of teasing and laughing and expressing tremendous joy. I am so blessed that I have him in my life at this point. He and my mother always taught me the importance of appreciating every moment in life, the importance of being present.

A few years ago, he fell and broke his hip. Here's a man who was in World War II, he was in a prisoner-of-war camp, he was active all his life. And I thought, Is this going to be it? Is he going to be so frustrated in that wheelchair that he won't be able to go on? No, not at all. I thought, Perhaps now is the time to refer him to hospice because I want to make sure I can manage things with him. I've taken a palliative-care approach with him for a number of years, but I want that additional level of support. If his symptoms get to the point at which he needs medication, I want to be able to handle his shortness of breath or pain while at the same time honoring his lifestyle. He's not used to a lot of medications.

D: Can you explain the difference between palliative care and hospice?

DR. P: Palliative care is a field of health-care medicine, an interdisciplinary field whose focus is on the care of the seriously and chronically ill. Then, as we get closer to a patient's death, palliative care can continue, but hospice is more of a designation recognizing that people may be in their last six months of life. I'm also a hospice medical codirector. I don't personally see a sharp demarcation between palliative care and hospice. What Medicare considers to be the criterion for hospice is a prognosis of six months or fewer. Medicare will also cover palliative care. It's a difference in time frame, but I think the approach is very similar.

D: Is medication offered during hospice and palliative care?

DR. P: In terms of managing physical symptoms and other symptoms, yes, absolutely.

D: I understand you've served in an advisory role with the Vatican. Tell me about that.

DR. P: The Vatican and the Pope, in particular, whom I love. Pope Francis is very supportive of palliative care and hospice. He delegated an advisory board to the Pontifical Academy for Life to explore palliative-care options globally. I had the tremendous honor and privilege to serve on the board for that initiative. We then had an international conference to discuss how the Church can support the development of palliative care worldwide. There's no question that the Vatican 100 percent supports palliative care. There's a tremendous need for all countries to develop it. People worldwide are suffering from all sorts of symptoms, including spiritual distress. Part of my role on the advisory committee was to talk about my work in interprofessional care and spiritual care, where we address spiritual distress. We work with specialists who are board-certified chaplains, health-care chaplains. In countries that don't have chaplains, there are other people who can fill the role of spiritual caregiver.

D: Given that background and the role you play there, I'd like to know how you feel about medical aid in dying.

DR. P: I'm concerned that in this society and in other countries where it's legal and where euthanasia is legal, I wonder what that says about our respect for life, for quality of life, for caring for people. When my patients request it, I ask them why, and what their concerns are. The concerns are, first, pain management and symptom management. Palliative care and hospice care can manage those. The next concern might be dignity, or lack thereof. "I don't want to be lying in bed, having people change my diapers." That's very real. I can tell you, however, that the people I've cared for, if that is done with respect for the individual — I think of how my dad's nurses change his diapers — it's an act of love and respect. I ask myself whether in the places where physician aid in dying is legal here in the States, in cultures and countries where euthanasia is legal, are we adversely affecting social norms? Are we giving a message that when you get to that point, there's not a lot of opportunity for meaning and purpose and joy?

D: As I understand, you did have a patient come to you and ask for medical aid in dying. Tell me about that experience and how you responded.

DR. P: I think that was one of the most moving experiences in my life, for the following reasons: I had promised this patient that I would be there to the end for her. That was our agreement and a deep, sacred part of my journey with her and my other patients. And when she asked me, in a flash I thought, Wait a minute, I promised to be there with her until the end and now she's asking me for something that I would find very difficult to do.

D: Do you remember her words?

DR. P: Not exactly. I think she said she wanted to explore how I felt about physician aid in dying, and whether in the course of her illness and eventual dying — she wasn't asking for the prescription at the time — I would be okay with writing the prescription for her. Before I answered, I wondered how I might honor my commitment to her to be present yet at the same time not do something that I am not comfortable with. So I told her that perhaps there are other physicians in my practice who are okay with writing these prescriptions and that I could refer her to another person when the time came. But I would still continue to be there with her. She did ask if I would be comfortable telling her why I have concerns. I usually try not to put my own beliefs out there, because I don't want the patient to be affected by my opinion. But in this case, I felt comfortable doing so. I shared with her my sense that, from my many experiences in caring for people as they approached death, if people were open to mystery and to the unknown, so many wonderful things might happen. Not that I want to sugarcoat the process.

But I felt that by taking a more medical approach, maybe the opportunity for the unexpected would be shut out. What if someone takes the medication, and then what if she hadn't and something good might have happened to her? I was very open about that with her. We agreed to disagree. It was a lovely conversation.

A few days before she died, I did a house call. I walked into her room and she was smiling and she said, "You were right." I asked her what she meant. And she talked about a very personal thing that had happened in her family that got resolved and said that maybe if she hadn't been here it might not have happened. And we just sat in silence in that moment. So while I understand it's legal and people can make the choices they need to make, what I would like to convey in this interview with you, Diane, is that we, as a culture, and particularly the baby boomers — we want control. I mean I do, too. We all do. We want to have our say. If we don't want to be in a nursing home, we don't want to be in a nursing home. I think making the process legal is one thing. I have some concerns about how it's being interpreted.

D: How do you feel about your colleagues who do physician aid in dying, who respond positively to people who are suffering from pain that palliative care cannot alleviate? Many palliative-care physicians acknowledge that there are times when it cannot relieve all the pain the patient is feeling.

DR. P: Different studies show that one of the main reasons for the request for aid in dying or euthanasia is actually spiritual or existential distress, and unfortunately, people often think there's nothing we can do for that. And I disagree. It's obviously an area I work in. I think we can address spiritual and existential distress. We're a very fix-it society, and so some of these questions about physician aid in dying have to do with a medical solution for these issues. There isn't a pill one can take for spiritual distress or existential distress. But I think that working with chaplains and other spiritual-care professionals can help alleviate that kind of distress.

There's a workforce issue in palliative care. My colleagues and all of us in health care are working in a system that increasingly asks more of us, placing a burden on the time we have. I think we need to ensure that every single palliative-care physician, nurse, chaplain, social worker has adequate time to fully address the suffering of a patient. I think the requests [for medical aid in dying] would decrease if my colleagues were given adequate support and staffing to be able to fully address patients' needs. I have no negative judgment about my colleagues who feel that [medical aid in dying] is in the best interest of their patients. But I haven't met a single colleague who feels totally comfortable with it. Even in states where it's legal and they write prescriptions for it, nobody is 100 percent comfortable with writing the prescriptions.

D: It's so interesting that in the twenty-two years that medical aid in dying has been legal in Oregon, one-third of the patients who've asked for and received the medication have not used it. They decided they'd rather go through the process, the journey, the mystery. But those other two-thirds have felt, as my husband did, that since he could no longer use his hands, he could no longer feed himself, stand on his own or toilet himself, that he had not only lost what he believed to be his dignity, but that he was no longer of use to society. He told my daughter, who is a physician, that he was ready to die, that he no longer had any joy in living. He had stopped reading, stopped watching television, and he slept most of the day.

Now I wonder whether his wish to die should not be taken as seriously spiritually as someone who agrees with you and wishes to plumb the mystery. Because John could not receive medical aid in dying, he had to starve himself and go without water or medication for ten days, until he died. I as his wife could do nothing but watch him suffer. And I could see that suffering on his face, though he never cried out. So I find myself wondering whether that desire for a physician's assistance is equally worthy of the honor of which you speak, as is the honor that one should receive as an older person, growing older and weaker.

DR. P: Thank you for sharing that very moving story, Diane. At some point in our life, we're all going to say, "I'm done and this is it." And absolutely, we should listen to that. I completely understand what you're saying, and part of me says, "Yes, when someone might be at that phase, what would be wrong with invoking that law?" But I think I'm looking at it not from the perspective of an individual case, but as an aspect of our culture and perhaps other cultures — a rise in loneliness and detachment. In health care, including in palliative care, it's even more prominent, where clinicians are stressed and overworked. What people desperately need is to be heard.

I wasn't privileged to be at the bedside of your husband or with you during that time, but when someone says something like that, Diane, "I'm done, I want to die," many clinicians unfortunately are not trained to sit and listen to the pain that is at the root of that statement. So they say they can't do anything about it, or they offer to write a prescription for conscious sedation. And that's a person's choice, it's legal. But are we forgetting about the other options? Are we overmedicalizing dying by saying, "Oh, you're at that point, so here, you can take these medications if you request them"? It may be the answer, for some. But I think another answer is to honor that time, to sit and listen and to train people to be present, to support families, to understand that the path isn't easy. Even taking those pills is not easy.

D: I want you to know the personal journey my husband went through. His doctor was very caring, and even in the care facility, he sat with John for long periods. He sat with John because he respected him and wanted to be of help to him, I think spiritually as well as physically. I am wondering whether you believe the American Medical Association is going to change its position on medical aid in dying as did the California Medical Association, the Oregon Medical Association, and Washington State. Three and perhaps other associations took a neutral stance, and that was their way of dealing with physician aid in dying. I wonder whether you see that happening at the AMA?

DR. P: I know that the position of neutrality for a number of organizations was well intended, in the sense that there are some physicians who are in favor of physician aid in dying and see it as a medical intervention. And there are many that are not. So these organizations are presenting physicians with both types of opinions. But it goes both ways. The physicians who are in favor of [aid in dying] are supported and are given adequate resources. But physicians who have ethical conflicts should also be supported, and not be pressured into support. I would hope that the AMA in its deliberations would look at what endorsing a law does to society.

D: And what do you think it does to society?

DR. P: I mentioned to you that I have spoken in countries where euthanasia is legal. I've had the opportunity to share fairly deeply with clinicians in those countries. I've heard stories. And I've seen in other countries, when people start saying, "I'm done with life, enough," they say that that's enough of a criterion to give them euthanasia. That's what I'm talking about. Do I think that might happen in this country? I don't know. I hope not. But the physicians I've been with or the nurses involved with cases like that, nobody is comfortable with it. I think the circumstances you described with your husband, I agree with you that there are times when all our medications may not help a person. But I also know that palliative sedation has been used, and I think it's been used effectively.

I know everything is done with a lot of caution and thought, and it's the same with physician aid in dying. But if it gets to the point that somehow our support of these new laws impacts the way we treat people toward the end of life, I would find that devastating. I hope that we have equal time for both conversations. Should physician aid in dying be allowed in all states? I would love to go back to that question. Have we lost the reverence for people in health-care systems, not just in end-of-life care?

D: Earlier, we talked about your being raised in the Roman Catholic Church, and your advisory role in that church. For you, then, does medical aid in dying truly violate everything that you believe in?

DR. P: That's a very personal question. I mean I can answer, in a sense that there's an assumption that because I'm a Catholic, I'm going to see something a certain way. I told you at the beginning of the interview that I actually have very broad beliefs, and very broad influences. First of all, the project that I was involved in with the Vatican is not just for the Church. It was actually a multifaith, as well as a secular, initiative. But you ask if this violates what as a Catholic I believe in. I'm a member of a secular order, Discalced Carmelites, and that's very important to me. But I've also been raised as a participant in many different faiths.

The question is, How do I, as a person of all my experiences, how do I feel? Does aid in dying violate my beliefs? *Violate* is a very, very strong word. I would not be able to write a prescription for someone that ended his or her life. And that's not because I'm Roman Catholic. It's because I'm Christina Puchalski, who was raised by a family who gave her the experience of loving life and valuing life and seeing the good in both suffering and joy, and that's accepting life. To be able to honor life in all its dimensions and not to have anyone feel that somehow they're less valuable because they're homeless or because they're dying or because they have their diapers changed or they can't stand up anymore, or walk or speak or think clearly. It's not a question of whether it violates my beliefs. It's more a hesitancy, a very strong concern I have that the law will somehow continue to perpetuate what I see as a social problem of the lack of dignity or the lack of respect for human life.

D: That's a beautiful answer. You talked about palliative care in the sense of dealing with the discomfort, the pain. I'm not talking here about spiritual pain, I'm talking about physical pain, but maybe I am also talking about spiritual pain. If I say to you that my physical pain is so great, my spiritual suffering is so great, that I cannot bear to live any longer, do I define my suffering for myself or does someone else define it for me?

DR. P: A person's suffering is their suffering. If you were my patient and you asked me that at the bedside, my response would be to listen. I would ask you to tell me more. I would try by doing a spiritual history, finding out what that spiritual distress or existential distress is about. I would want to know more about social disconnectedness, feeling isolated. And I would certainly do a full assessment for your physical pain and symptoms, and offer you the things I could to help you, not to fix you.

D: When I die, I want to be awake. I want to have my family with me. I do not want to be so sedated that I do not know they are with me. I want to hug them and kiss them and tell them how much they mean to me. I wonder what your own idea of a good death would be.

DR. P: I don't actually believe in that concept of a "good" death. I don't have any expectations, because I have learned from my own life, and from making this journey with others, that people change. We don't always know what we want, and this gets back to our generation of wanting to control everything. What you say today, what I say today, may not be what we say when we are facing our deaths. When it really comes down to it, I don't know what I'm going to say. You don't know what you're going to say. We need to be open.

D: I guess it's what I would wish for.

DR. P: Yes. There's such freedom when people let go of these plans, and such joy that can come into their lives. I would love for us to just be present in the moment to everybody, and to ourselves in particular. And be open to where our lives may turn.

DAN DIAZ

WIDOWER OF BRITTANY MAYNARD

In 2007, Dan Diaz met the woman who was to become his wife. Brittany had just graduated from the University of California, Berkeley. In contrast to what he calls his own "more grounded, stable, sturdy" personality, Brittany had a sense of adventure. After their first date, it didn't take long for them to decide they were a couple. Brittany grew up in Southern California and had always enjoyed the beach, surf, and sand. Then during her early twenties, her gaze shifted to the mountains, and she really came to love living in Boulder, Colorado.

Brittany summited Kilimanjaro and Cotopaxi. She worked in an orphanage in Southeast Asia for six months. When Dan and Brittany married, in September 2012, they honeymooned in Patagonia and hiked glaciers.

I began by asking Dan to tell me when he

and Brittany started to realize she was having health problems.

DAN: A few months after our wedding, she started having headaches. They would wake her up in the middle of the night. She would get sick and then be unable to get back to sleep. That lasted for a few months. She wasn't losing weight and her appetite wasn't decreasing; it was just the headaches. She went to see a specialist, who didn't order a CT scan. When she described her symptoms, he said she was probably going through light sensitivity, sensitivity to loud sounds, and a few other things that made him believe they were migraines and nothing more.

In 2013, the headaches went away by the summer, and she was feeling okay. But by the end of the year, they started coming back. During those holidays in particular, and on New Year's Eve, when we were in wine country on a trip that Brittany had planned for us, the pain was just getting too intense and something seemed horribly wrong. We went to the emergency room, and the physician in

Healdsburg, California, ordered a CT scan.

And that was when we discovered the tumor and the size of it. Most physicians who saw it said it was one of the biggest tumors they'd ever seen.

DIANE: Did the doctor suggest surgery to try to remove the tumor as a whole?

DAN: Yes. Unfortunately there was no cure, only certain treatment options, the first one being surgery. So ten days later, on January 10, Brittany underwent an eight-hour brain surgery at the University of California, San Francisco Medical Center. They were only able to remove about 35 to 40 percent of the tumor — because of the size and location of it, that's all they could safely get. At that point, they informed Brittany that three to five years of life was all the time she had left.

D: And what would have happened had they gone further and tried to remove more of the tumor?

DAN: There are certain parts of the brain that the surgeons said they just couldn't get into, that the person will not wake up from surgery, or may end up in a vegetative state. And also the way the tumor was diffused: it had worked its way into many different parts of the brain that a surgeon's knife or scalpel cannot get into. The damage that would be caused might end up killing the person instead of saving her.

D: How long did it take for Brittany to recuperate after the operation?

DAN: That was actually surprisingly quick. She was back at home within three or four days. I remember that evening in the intensive care unit, after she had come out of surgery she was still groggy, but talking to her, and her to me, that was such a relief, just hearing her voice, hearing her describing what she was feeling to the nurses. They said she should get up and move around. Her recovery was within two weeks.

I mentioned that the prognosis was three to five years. But just two months later, the first follow-up MRI showed signs that the tumor was growing aggressively, which was indicative of a glioblastoma multiforme. That's the most aggressive type of brain cancer. At that point, they informed Brittany that six months was all the time she had left. So it went from three or five years to, all of a sudden, six months.

That was just devastating to her, to us. We were at that point planning on starting a family, so the idea that her life would now be cut short when she was twenty-nine years old . . . it took a while to process that. It was a few days of just wanting to be with one another and process the reality of what we'd just heard, the enormity of that tumor . . . it was just devastating to all of us.

D: Were any decisions made between the two of you at the time, as you processed that news?

DAN: Before she went into surgery, Brittany was researching different treatment options, clinical trials that might be available to her. She had already found the Oregon Death with Dignity program. In her undergrad time at UC Berkeley, that topic was discussed in one of her classes. For me it was brand new. I was unaware that such a program even existed. So, by January 3 or 4, Brittany told me we would continue to fight this tumor. "But if shit gets bad," she said, "we're moving to Oregon." She knew how that brain tumor would end her life, and it would be a brutal dying process, so she simply wanted to have peace of mind that her final few days "on this green earth," as she said, her dying process, would be gentle, and that she would not suffer horrifically. By the end of the conversation, I recognized that, if I were in her position, I would be saying the exact same thing. There wasn't any sort of conversation of her trying to convince me — it was just kind of automatic, like, of course, that's what we will do.

D: So Brittany brought up the idea that you and she would move to Oregon from California?

DAN: Yeah, and those details are what we worked through. Based on the research that she went on doing, she found that she would have to become a resident of Oregon, which meant she would have to get a driver's license and change her voter registration. We'd have to rent a house, and she found a house to rent on Craigslist. She found a new medical team at Oregon Health & Science University. She went through all those steps and decided to speak up because she thought it was a huge injustice that a terminally ill individual, after being told she had six months to live, all of a sudden had to go through the process of leaving her home to get across some imaginary line on a map; that in Oregon, she would have the option of a gentle passing, but that if we stayed in California, she ran the risk of essentially being tortured to death by the brain tumor.

D: Dan, I'm wondering about the practicalities here. What about your job, your ability to earn a living? What about the practicalities of moving to Oregon?

DAN: None of it was easy. I ended up having to take a leave of absence from work, and when that occurs, of course, your salary gets adjusted down. I think it was you get 60 percent of your salary, and then you have to contribute more to certain benefits and health insurance, so it took a lot of orchestrating and talking to Human Resources. When I look back at the fact that we had to go through that process, having to go through the bureaucracy and getting all this taken care of, that's the time we felt cheated of and wanted back. Brittany also knew there are so many people who would not have the resources and ability to do this. I'm thirteen years older than Brittany, and I had worked very hard to get us somewhat established, and the idea that we were paying a mortgage in California and also the rental of a house in Oregon, maintaining two properties, and paying electrical bills times two — no, nobody should have to go through that. That's why Brittany spoke up.

D: I know this is not easy, and I don't want to make you uncomfortable. Are you okay talking with me about all of this?

DAN: Oh sure. Sharing Brittany's story is the promise that I made to her.

D: It's Brittany's story, but it's also your story, because you were left behind. You know, there is a coincidence here because I go out to OHSU for my voice treatments. It's a wonderful place, and I'm glad you and she had that kind of institutional care.

DAN: Her palliative-care team at OHSU truly was extraordinary. It provided the support she needed to navigate the six months while we were up there in Portland.

D: So at that time, Brittany was a resident of the state of Oregon, and you remained a resident of the state of California? Going back and forth while she was there, or staying with her the whole time?

DAN: There were certain things that Brittany wanted to do with the time she had left, which included traveling to certain destinations. One of the places we went to was Yellowstone National Park, where she'd wanted to go for quite a while. When we were on that trip, in May, we received an e-mail saying that Brittany was approved for secobarbital, the medication used for medical aid in dying. By July, we were both in Oregon full-time. I ended up taking a six-month leave of absence from work.

D: And was Brittany experiencing pain during that time?

DAN: She felt a lot of pressure at the base of her skull and neck. From February to May, things were better — she wasn't in pain too much of the time. But by July, August, September, October . . . those last two months she was getting more and more uncomfortable. The seizures were what terrified her the most, and those became more frequent and more severe. I could often tell a seizure was happening before she would notice it because I would see her left eyelid start to flutter. And she said she had a metallic taste in her mouth. A seizure happens when electrical impulses in a person's brain are firing, and it makes the muscles in that person's body twitch and contract. The expression on her face became different because her muscles were contracting. The rest of her body would start to twitch — her arms, her legs — and we'd typically get her sitting. A few happened while we were standing, while we were on a hike, and she would quickly sit down and I would be there to support her. She would usually be unable to speak or communicate at all or to write anything for maybe twenty to thirty minutes afterward. The sentences she would try to form just wouldn't make any sense.

Those were the mild seizures. The full grand mal seizures, where every muscle in her body was contracting, were terrifying since on a couple of occasions, as she came out of the seizure and kind of regained consciousness, blood came out of her mouth because

82

she'd bitten through part of her tongue. My job was just to keep her from being injured by an external object or by falling and hitting the ground. Twice she was near a bed, so she managed to get to the bed and I managed to keep her from falling off it as her body went through those convulsions.

D: Were those convulsions part of the reason she made the decision that the time was coming close?

DAN: The seizures certainly played a part in tracking the progression of the tumor. There were days when she would say, "Today I can tell, it feels like I am dying." The inability to sleep for days on end, the vomiting, the seizures, these are the things she was sort of using to gauge the progression of the tumor. And in addition, we had monthly MRI scans where we could see the progression of the tumor.

D: Between those seizures, did she experience happiness? Did she experience an ability to enjoy life, even if only for brief periods?

DAN: Yes. Thanks to her determination, Brittany kept on taking trips. We went to Olympic National Park in Washing-

83

ton, we went to the Columbia River District in Oregon. We took a helicopter tour of the Grand Canyon. That was during the last two weeks of Brittany's life. These were the things she wanted to do as she was fighting against that tumor, battling in order to enjoy the things that were so important to her.

D: Did the fact that she had been approved to receive the drug she wanted to use to end her life somehow give her freedom to enjoy what she had left, because she knew when her moment came, she had the power to end her suffering?

DAN: When she received approval for the medication, it provided her an enormous sense of relief, a sense of having just a little bit of control in the midst of the chaos of a brain tumor. So much felt completely out of her control. Having the secobarbital allowed her to focus on life, because she no longer had to be so concerned about the dying process. It allowed her to do the things she wanted to do. It was very evident to me how much relief it provided her. Her outlook from that point on was completely different.

That fear was gone. She could now focus on living life, not being so terrified of death.

D: Brittany chose November 1, 2014, to end her life. She chose that publicly, weeks in advance. Can you tell me why?

DAN: I think people will understand. Brittany wanted to live to celebrate two dates in particular. One was our wedding anniversary, which is September 29. To get through that month of September, she was really battling against the symptoms as she was feeling the cancer continuing to grow. The second date that Brittany wanted to celebrate was my birthday, October 26. So she said that if she possibly could, she'd try to make it to November 1.

By no means was that any sort of a hard-and-fast date. Brittany set herself the goal to celebrate those two special days. I asked one of her physicians about this, whether terminally ill patients sometimes set these goals. And the doctor said, "Oh yeah, some patients absolutely do." They say, "I want to live to this date," and if they achieve that, they'll set another one. But in

October, things started getting much worse.

The pain became more and more intense. She would sleep with this heating pad around her neck because of the pressure at the base of her skull. It was like this beanbag, and we would have to heat it up in the microwave, and then she would put it there. It would feel good for a while, and she'd be able to get a little bit of sleep. But sleep became a luxury.

During the last month of her life, the seizures were coming every four or five days. As the tumor continued to grow and put pressure on different parts of the brain, it would push on the optic nerve and she would lose her eyesight. It's not uncommon for a person who has a brain tumor to suffer a stroke. Depending on what part of the brain is damaged due to lack of oxygen during the stroke, that person can lose the ability to stand, walk, swallow, the ability to communicate altogether. Partial paralysis was likely, complete paralysis was a possibility. That's what Brittany was facing. And she said, "I will not die that way."

The biggest safeguard of medical aid

in dying is that two physicians, independent of each other, have to agree that this person is terminally ill, that she has six months or less to live, and that she is mentally competent. The patient must make the request both orally and in writing. There's a fifteen-day waiting period, and there are witnesses involved. Another strong safeguard is that the individual has to be able to consume the medication on her own. So, if Brittany waits too long, or if she does suffer a stroke, it leaves her trapped in her own body and she's unable to consume that medication. She would end up dying the very way she was trying to avoid, suffering a massive stroke in bed with tubes coming out of her. That's the thought process Brittany was going through, making decisions based on what she was suffering day after day and the progress we were seeing from those MRIs. So it did end up being November 1.

D: Can you tell me about that day, how it began? The press was very much focused on it. I felt so horrible for her as we in the public were watching this poor young woman suffering through this horrendous problem, making her decision in public. I wanted to know about the private side.

DAN: In one regard, rest assured that Brittany and I did not feel that pressure or that we were under a microscope as far as the public was concerned. That was family time, and we were taking care of one another. She released a video at that time, saying the decision was hers, that it should rest with the terminally ill individual. The hope is that you don't need to use the medication, but the decision belongs to that individual, and that's a good thing.

Well, the media ran with the story, because she said that if she were still alive on November 2, it just meant we were navigating through this. It must have been a slow news day. Somebody said, "Oh, now this girl has changed her mind from November 1 to November 2." And that's bullshit. There was no story there. They took Brittany's words out of context, spun them into something they wanted to, and ran with that story. Shame on them. That's not what you asked about, but just so you know, that's what was going on from our point of view.

As far as November 1, my wife was a bit of a planner. She had laid out a lot of instructions for me, pertaining to the ceremony she wanted, where to scatter her ashes, how she wanted that ceremony to go. She had instructions for some of her friends, instructions certainly for me, about the dogs, and things pertaining to our house. So on November 1, Brittany had her friends there at the house in Portland, and she said she wanted to go for a hike that morning. We went for a walk because by then she wasn't feeling that great. Her parents, three of her friends, one of my younger brothers, and the two dogs. We walked Brittany's favorite trail.

I want to be clear that there wasn't this sense of a heavy, dark feeling or anything. It was just a conversation about life and love and fun times. We were probably gone from the house for close to two hours.

Brittany had had a small seizure that morning. It was a reminder of what she was risking. When we got back to the house, she told me, "It's my time." That's what she said. There are other details that I do want to keep personal and private.

D: I understand.

DAN: She had time with each of us, with her friends, going through certain things from her closet, giving certain things to her friends. And there's a process regarding the medication. The patient first takes something that gets the system ready so there are no issues in the stomach.

D: To keep it there, and not to expel it.

DAN: Exactly. And since this was all at Brittany's direction and she was controlling the whole process, I think that's why there wasn't any anxiety. There were one hundred capsules. One of Brittany's friends and my younger brother opened them. I helped out with some of that, but I wanted to be next to Brittany during all this time. Brittany's mother and her stepdad, Gary, were next to her beside the bed. Her friends were at the foot of the bed. And Brittany said, "I want people to be comfortable, so we'll have chairs so people can sit or they can stand if they want." And I was in bed next to her and we actually had our small dog, Bella the Beagle, in bed with us as well. It was a very loving feeling. And she said she wanted us to talk about happy things. So she was in bed and I was next to her in the bed, with her friends surrounding her.

The secobarbital, after it's prepared, has to be mixed with about four or five ounces of water. Within five minutes after consuming it, she fell asleep, and it's just as if a person is being sedated, she gets groggy and little by little, falls asleep, no different from the thousands of times I'd seen Brittany fall asleep during the seven-plus years I knew her. I was tracking her breathing, and at around thirty minutes it continued to lessen, and it slowed to the point where Brittany passed away. That was the dying process.

D: So peaceful.

DAN: And that's not at all how her dying process would have gone if the brain tumor had continued to run its course and inflict all of those horrific symptoms on her, the seizures, the pain, the nausea, the vomiting, and what was coming, which was right around the corner, the likelihood of blindness or paralysis.

It's not that Brittany was choosing between living and dying. The living part was not on the table. The only thing Brittany was choosing between was two different ways of dying. One was gentle, the other would have been filled with pain and suffering. It's something that I try to emphasize because I think people have the wrong frame of mind. She wanted to live. The brain tumor was ending her life.

D: Dan, you and I have both been speaking around the country about medical aid in dying. I have heard so many people raise the question of religious belief as a reason not to end one's own life despite the suffering. I believe that if someone feels God should be the only taker of life, I respect that, and I'm sure you do, too. How do you respond to those who say no one should be allowed to take one's life no matter what?

DAN: With full respect for an individual who, if they were in Brittany's predicament, would wish to attempt to pray away the pain, pray away those seizures, pray away that advancing brain tumor, I'd be the first one to defend their decision to make sure their wishes are carried out. The strength of this program [medical aid in dying] is that it's an option that a person has to apply for, qualify for, and finally be granted. If for religious reasons, somebody in Brittany's predicament is not on board, then they simply wouldn't apply for it.

Curiously enough, though, a poll done by a Christian organization shows that support among Christians is just about 70 percent. Support among Catholics is 70 percent. I was in Massachusetts, where good old Irish Catholics in Boston at the State House supported it by 72 percent. In New York, even though the council of bishops is opposed to it, support among Catholics is closer to 74 percent.

While I understand the official position of the institution of the Catholic Church, the congregants agree with Brittany, that a terminally ill individual should have the option of medical aid in dying. And since I grew up Catholic, I know I frustrate them because I have absolutely no problem reconciling this medical practice with my faith and my relationship with God. God is a loving, caring, compassionate deity, and there's no conflict there at all for me. It just comes down to the individual.

D: Do you see the country moving in the direction that you and Brittany chose, and do you believe greater acceptance is coming?

DAN: I think so. When Brittany died, there were four states that allowed medical aid in dying: Oregon, Washington, Vermont, and Montana. In the last two and a half years since Brittany died, we've passed legislation in California, Colorado, D.C., New Jersey, and Maine. I have to remind myself that legislative matters move slowly, but I'm impatient.

I do believe that Brittany's story made a huge impact on passing legislation in California, Colorado, and D.C. But opposition to this legislation, even in states that have passed it, continues. Quite regularly, some lawsuit will be brought by an attorney who's representing maybe one or two physicians as plaintiffs. This happens in Oregon, Montana, California. For twenty years, the opposition has tried to chip away at the legislation or use a different angle in the attempt to get it overturned or negated. But that's where an organization like Compassion & Choices comes in. They send attorneys to battle against that. So the opposition will continue in its efforts, but the good news is that the law has been in effect for twenty years in Oregon and the plaintiffs have been unsuccessful.

D: I've been told that some doctors refuse to refer a dying patient to a physician who is participating in medical aid in dying. That seems pretty awful to me.

DAN: Yes, to the point that some physicians refuse to recommend a dying patient to a prescribing physician or a participating physician. That is frustrating.

D: Finally, Dan, how are you?

DAN: Not a day goes by that I don't think about Brittany and reflect on what our life was like. I miss that girl. It's been two and a half years, and I still think about her, even now in moments like this, when I'm with my family, on vacation. I still think, She's not here with us to be a part of this. But she was explicit with me, saying I needed to do the things she and I had wanted to do, to eventually have a family and to continue little projects she and I had talked about around the house. Brittany was trying to make it easier for me in my grieving process, and it's something I am ever grateful for. I loved Brittany with all my heart, and she loved me that same way. There's a quote I found that I tend to keep at the top of my mind: "You can cry that it's over, or you can smile that it happened."

MARTHA KAY NELSON

DIRECTOR OF SPIRITUAL CARE AT
MISSION HOSPICE & HOME CARE

Martha Kay Nelson has had a long career in hospice work. Rather than choosing hospice work, she believes hospice work chose her. Her training was at Harvard Divinity School. She did a yearlong internship as a hospice chaplain during her graduate work. The year after she graduated, she managed to combine her career as a chaplain with her work in hospice. She is in her mid-forties, with short hair and hazel eyes. Her warm, open face, earnest manner, and easy smile help me understand why she is so good at her work. We sit together in her office at Mission Hospice & Home Care in San Mateo, California.

DIANE: How do you feel about California's "right to die" law?
MARTHA: Well, I have many feelings, and they could vary depending on the day or the hour. It depends on whom

I'm talking to, and what her or his experience is. My overall sense about the law is that people have a right to make their own health-care decisions, whether it's at the end of life or at any time up to that point. I know people have a hard time having these conversations, particularly early on, before they're even sick. And then they get sick and it's crisis time, and those decisions have to be made quickly. The End of Life Option Act to me is part of a spectrum of all those decisions and conversations that come at the end. It's a new end point on that spectrum.

D: You've been in a leadership position here at Mission Hospice, not only learning, but teaching. Tell me what have been the elements of transmitting this information to others.

M: It's been an interesting learning curve. I think even seasoned hospice professionals have had to adjust to a new option for patients, stepping into that terrain. The elements that have been important in teaching staff members, working with health-care partners, have been to get folks to acknowledge at the outset that this is a challenging topic, this is new terrain, there are profound implications, and not to shy away from it.

Some folks here at Mission Hospice didn't want to participate, but the majority did, to have their questions answered or share some of their thoughts, their concerns. We've done this regularly enough that people felt they could talk freely about the End of Life Option Act. We didn't want it to be whispered about awkwardly in the corner, that this law is coming and our patients are going to have the right to choose the option. As an agency, we're not advocates for the law, we're advocates for our patients, and we won't abandon them. Having said that, any of our employees, if they're not comfortable, don't have to participate. They can opt out if they need to, and they would be fully supported.

D: What kinds of questions did you get from staff? What kinds of issues did they raise?

M: At the outset, a lot of general questions about details of the law, how it works, how are we supposed to communicate with our colleagues around it, what can we say to the patient and what can't we, those kinds of things. Questions arose about accessibility to the law. If I have patients who are saying they just want to end it all, and they're saying this a lot, but they're not specifically asking about the law, then can I bring it up with them or not? We have a policy here at Mission Hospice that we let the patient lead. If a patient is inquiring about his or her options, then we will be there.

That's one kind of question. Other clinicians have asked about folks who haven't had the chance to be educated about medical aid in dying, or don't have access to resources where they might have learned about it. What if it's something they'd like to avail themselves of? There's kind of a social justice question there. There are also questions arising from specific cases. Every case is different.

D: Can you give me an idea of how many patients have actually come forward and asked you about the right to die?

M: We've been tracking some of these numbers, and to date, we've served around forty-five people since California's law went into effect, which was a lot more than we anticipated. When back in 2016 we set out to draft our policy and prepare ourselves, we thought maybe we'd have four or five people in the first year. We had twenty-one. And about that same number inquired about the law, but never went all the way through the process. Either they actually died before they had a chance to use the law, or they changed their minds. I would imagine that it was split evenly.

D: Tell me about the process. So a patient comes to you and asks about the process, the law. How do you respond?

M: My initial response as a chaplain would be one of curiosity. I'd be interested in learning more about their thoughts and why they're asking. It's a big thing to ask about. Sometimes people are afraid to even inquire. They're afraid of being shamed or judged. So I'd want to let that person know that I'm glad they're asking. And then we'd have a conversation, whatever they would wish to say at that time. Next, I would contact the doctor and the rest of my interdisciplinary team members and would let them know the topic had been broached. Then a doctor would probably go and make a direct visit, which would be considered the first formal request, if the decision was made to pursue that course.

We really encourage the other team members to make sure they keep talking to one another — the social worker, the nurse, the spiritual counselor, home health aides, and volunteers who might also be involved. Through a team effort, we would need to have clarity on how much privacy the patient would want. Patients have the right under the law to not tell anyone but the doctors they're working with, not even family members. Our experience has been that that's not often the case. Usually there is communication with family.

D: Who makes the initial judgment that the patient has six months or less to live?

M: The attending physician on the case. And if the patient inquires about the law, and his or her doctor says, "I'm not comfortable being involved with this," that's one way we might get involved. Or it might be a hospice patient already on our service.

D: I saw in your waiting room a brochure for Death Cafes. Can you tell me about them?

M: The Death Cafe movement started several years ago in England. It's basically having a conversation over coffee and cakes in a public venue. Anyone is welcome to attend, and the purpose is open-ended. The goal is to talk about death in any way you wish. There does need to be a facilitator, someone who is able to establish ground rules in etiquette so folks aren't talking over one another. Folks that host them tend to have some level of experience in end-of-life care, in thanatology, but anyone can sign up. I've led a couple of them.

D: How successful do you think Death Cafes are as teaching tools, as comforting elements in the whole discussion of death?

M: I think Death Cafes are successful in meeting the needs of folks who already want to talk about death. If you show up at a Death Cafe, there's something in you that is already ready to speak and to hear what other people are thinking. It can serve as a cross-pollination of ideas and thoughts, and normalization. The cafes meet a kind of thirst that we have in our culture to speak about these things openly and not be afraid. How you get people to Death Cafes is another question. I've had some people say they're offended by that name, or they don't want to attend a Death Cafe because it sounds morbid.

D: What is the best way to reach people? How do we get the conversation started even before we're sick?

M: There's no one best way. It's about being creative and really getting to know your community. In my family, I've been lucky in that we've always talked about death openly. I have ongoing conversations now with my father. He's about to turn eighty-three, and I really value the kinds of discussions and ruminations we have.

It's wonderful. We've started kind of reflecting theologically, talking about, wondering together, what happens after we die. To be able to have that in a father-daughter kind of way. I'm well aware of what a precious opportunity it is to hear his thoughts. As he comes into the "lean and slippered pantaloon" time of his life, as he might say — some of his last chapters — I feel really blessed that he's willing to discuss it openly.

D: How do you open that discussion for the general public?

M: I think it takes courage and a conscious decision to ask a question of someone in a moment when you feel there's an opportunity. Someone speaking about her or his health, some decline, or illness, grief, and you ask, "How would you like things to be?" And perhaps even being a bit persistent if you get an initial brush-off, which often happens, but trying again, and saying, "Really, I would like to know."

I also think reaching children is important. I think that in our death-denying culture, children are really shielded from all things involved with death. Things happen at the funeral parlor, no longer at home, and we try to protect children in all kinds of ways. But if you don't allow children who want to be involved in a loved one's illness or death, I think you're doing them a disservice. You're keeping them from something that is integral to life for all of us. The earlier you can start to have those experiences and wonder about them and ask the questions, the more skills you will have as you age to meet them openly.

D: Have you decided what you want for yourself at the end?

M: I have no idea. I do know that I would like to have the right and the option to choose. I understand that even just knowing that the option is available can bring a lot of comfort to people. I haven't faced a terminal illness that might cause me great physical pain or suffering, or mental or spiritual suffering. There's one area that gives me pause, which is when folks choose medical aid in dying because they're used to being in control in their lives. They might not have physical or mental or spiritual suffering, but they want to have personal agency. I think they entirely have the right to do that. But I also believe we're in a culture that distorts the degree to which we think we're in control. So on a soul level, on a much deeper level, I wonder, Are we messing with something there? How is it that we're making such a profound decision from a place of a distorted need for control? And then I think, Well, what do I know about their journey and what they need? Maybe this is the one time they've ever made a strong, solid decision for themselves, and who am I to say what it is they need to learn?

D: But isn't pain, intractable pain and suffering, and the inability to care for oneself, a sufficient reason to respect someone's decision in terms of his or her final say?

M: Absolutely. I think clinicians have more trouble when they can't observe visible intractable pain, when they can't see physical or emotional suffering. It's harder for clinicians to get their heads and hearts around that. Why is someone making this choice? And so I do a lot of counseling with staff about that, exploring how to meet the needs of the person when we don't see them suffering, at least not on the surface. And we have to remind ourselves, clinicians need to express those feelings and concerns, so that when they're dealing with patients directly, they can be respectful and meet them on their own terms.

HEATHER MASSEY

DEATH EDUCATOR

I met with Heather Massey at the First Congregational Church of the United Church of Christ in Falmouth, Massachusetts. It's a lovely old New England church, typical of those in the area, with a tall white steeple, a clock, stained glass windows, and old wooden pews. Heather is the facilitator for the Cape Cod Death Cafe, and identifies herself as a death educator. We're seated in an area outside the main chapel furnished with comfortable sofas and chairs. She sips a glass of water as she tells me about her background in medical social work, as an administrator in both clinical hospital and hospice settings.

DIANE: How did you become a "death educator"?

HEATHER: I've been involved with helping to teach people about death and the concerns of the dying for most of my life. In the last ten years in particular, since the death of my mother, I've been very involved in the home death care movement. I teach families how to care for their loved ones, as well as being a consumer advocate, working on alternatives for people regarding final disposition, burial at sea, green burial, et cetera.

D: Tell me about Death Cafes and your involvement.

H: About six years ago, I heard about the Death Cafes that had just started in England. The very first ones, called *cafés mortels,* were actually in Switzerland, started by a Swiss sociologist. Then Jon Underwood, an artist who does a lot of different installations under the term "Impermanence," and his mother, Sue Reid, heard about them, and they started offering a Death Cafe in Jon's home in England. It was very popular, people asked them to come to their homes, and it spread in England. Then Jon and Sue got together and created the DeathCafe.com website, and a manual on how to host a Death Cafe elsewhere, because they realized they had hit on something that's a real need in our culture.

D: Did you get to meet Jon Underwood?

H: I never got to meet him in person, but I did do a training with him via teleconference. He did that with Americans who wanted to do it.

D: He must be a fascinating fellow.

H: He was. He just died this summer [2017], at forty-four, totally unexpectedly. He died with a completely undiagnosed congenital condition they were unaware of. There was an incident, and then he was gone. It's interesting that he was so attracted to helping people embrace life and death and the importance of death, and that he exited so soon himself. He was a remarkable young man. His mother, Sue, and his sister, Jools, are both carrying on the Death Cafe website and helping to promote the movement in general because it's worldwide now.

D: Tell me how Jon Underwood's work evolved into what's happening here in this country.

H: When I did training with Jon, I really wanted to bring that to Massachusetts and have this in our communities. At a Death Cafe, people talk about anything to do with the dying process, after death, funerals, all sorts of things.

There's no place in our culture where we can go and have those kinds of discussions. So it's really filled a void, and despite what the end-of-life options are or not here in Massachusetts, there are still people who want to explore them. It empowers them to ask questions about what is available to them or their loved ones, and gives them an opportunity to gain some knowledge as well.

D: Do people who are sick come to these Death Cafes looking for assistance?

H: Yes. We do stress that it's not a bereavement group and it's not a support group for those who are dying, but we do have all kinds of people who come. And they're looking for a place to share what they're experiencing.

D: You hold these Death Cafes once a month. Do you select a particular topic?

H: We don't choose topics. One of the principles of Death Cafe is that you don't lead anybody in any one direction or to any course of action or conclusion. It is group led. So whoever shows up at any given Death Cafe brings certain topics to the table. The facilitator has each person introduce himself or herself, to get a sense of what people would like to talk about and initiate the conversation.

D: How do you choose facilitators?

H: We've been very fortunate here. I like people who've had some form of training. We have two physicians, we have a therapist, we have a newspaper editor, and we have a minister amongst our regular facilitators. We meet regularly and talk about how everything is going.

D: Is there a bias in any of the discussions toward assisted suicide?

H: We don't call it "assisted suicide," Diane. Is there a bias toward that? Here's what I'd like to say about medical aid in dying. While it's not a topic deliberately chosen for discussion at Death Cafe, it has come up from the very beginning and it doesn't stop. That, and voluntary stopping of eating and drinking is another topic that comes up. One way of lessening the fear of death is to have some control over the uncontrollable, and to be able to discuss what those fears are and to know that there are options and choices. That comes up every single time.

D: I know you've worked with Roger Kligler. Tell me how that relationship came about and how you've worked together.

H: Roger and I met three years ago, in this very location. Roger and Cathy, his wife, came to a Death Cafe and death education program. It was the largest crowd we'd had — 120 people. The topic was medical aid in dying in Massachusetts. We also had Marie Manis, the chairperson of the Massachusetts chapter of Compassion & Choices. Despite the cold that night, so many people came because they were eager to learn what was being proposed in changes to the law. Roger came up to me and said, "I want to be involved in your Death Cafe, and I'd like to be involved with death education and Compassion & Choices, so who do I talk to?" He and I became fast friends, working together. We like to take our show on the road.

D: Did he tell you of his condition? [Roger has prostate cancer.]

H: Not initially. But he did tell me about it before he started talking more openly at the tables and with the folks who come to our programs.

113

D: Are there others who've come to the Death Cafe and said, "You know, I'm really sick. And I've been told I have a limited time to live, and I want to know what my options are"?

H: Yes, they want a place to come and talk about it. Some people can't talk with their families or haven't learned how to talk with their families, and coming to Death Cafe helps them learn some of those communications skills or approaches. Sometimes we do talk about how difficult it can be to speak to family members about it.

D: What about young people? Do they come, as well as older folks?

H: Yes, but not as many. The majority of our participants are probably baby boomers, reaching that point where they've begun thinking about what lies ahead. Or they have aging parents.

D: I have the impression that this whole movement is truly catching on across the country, and that people are thinking about what happens when they die, and how to prepare. I think that's fairly new because we're living longer.

H: I think when we realize that we're all going to die, and we think about death and the opportunities there are, it enhances our lives to be able to embrace it as an important part of life, just as important as birth.

D: Do the people who come to Death Cafes want to be educated, for example about voluntary stopping of eating and drinking?

H: We make it pretty clear, because we've agreed to be part of the social franchise that is Death Cafe, not to do education at the tables. So we created the death education program as something that is separate but meets the need, because the majority of people who come want to learn. They want to know what their options are. But in terms of lecturing or talking about action options, we reserve that for our programs.

D: Tell me why you think these end-of-life discussions are so important.

H: It's an important part of life that has been hidden for so long. It's been a taboo subject, and we don't have an opportunity to talk about death and dying. Death is hidden away. Death now happens generally in a hospital or a facility, or behind closed doors. We don't interact with the dying, and so it's unfamiliar. I think that's where the fear comes from: death just doesn't seem normal. Only a few decades ago, Grandpa used to die at home, and the family cared for him and maybe his body afterward. We've hidden ourselves from death. It's important to bring it out of the closet, to hold conversations. Talking about death can be a life-affirming exercise.

Rev. William Lamar

METROPOLITAN AFRICAN METHODIST EPISCOPAL CHURCH, WASHINGTON, D.C.

Reverend Lamar and I meet in the sanctuary of the Metropolitan AME Church. The balcony railings are covered with African kente cloths of every color. The curved wooden pews are original to the building, strong, sturdy, in an arena-like formation, and magnificently sculpted at each end. Stained glass windows are on both sides of the interior, with a large pipe organ at the front. At the back of the church is a large round stained glass window, which reminds me of the rose window at the back of the Washington National Cathedral.

I ask Reverend Lamar about the church.

REV. LAMAR: This church was completed in the 1880s. If you consider that time, and persons of African descent building a facility this grand . . . I tell people that it speaks to the fact that they viewed themselves and they viewed their God very differently than society viewed them. And they wanted their progeny to see themselves as large, to see their accomplishments as large, and to trust that there was a God who would help them in that quest.

In the 1880s, African Americans could not participate broadly in the larger economy. So they had to self-finance the structure. When you look around and you read the inscriptions in the windows, you'll see Georgia Conference, Alabama, Texas, Tennessee. All of the localities where there are African Methodists throughout the nation sent money so the church could be built. And if you sent, I believe, a hundred dollars, you got the name of your conference on a window. So these windows tell the story of persons, some of whom might have been enslaved, most probably the children of enslaved, who gathered meager resources. I often want to talk about the fact that these persons were philanthropists. We normally think of philanthropists as persons with access to huge resources. But these were true philanthropists. They took meager resources, pooled them together, and were able to build not only stunning churches but amazing universities and colleges and institutions that shielded life in the midst of much of America's brutality in that period.

Turning to another subject, I said I believed he had opposed the passage of the District of Columbia's medical aid in dying law.

REV. L: Yes. Diane, the reason I opposed the law was the deep history of malfeasance when it comes to the United States of America and the medical establishment's lack of commitment to caring equally for bodies that are not white. I feel like it's my responsibility to not take at face value things that are said about what we will do, how we will enforce equity, because there are just too many examples of those things not happening.

There are some things that are as American as apple pie, and that kind of inequity is very American. I don't know if at the macrolegislative level those things can be addressed. They have to be addressed person by person, case by case. I think it's a matter of understanding the spirit and intent of the law, but being very cautious about how the law itself is interpreted and executed. If the world were filled with people like you, I might feel differently. But I'm also aware, based on history and current events, that those things don't often happen. Support for this law could be used in a backdoor way to injure the very people that I seek to assist. I feel like I'm playing a politician's game right now, and I really don't want to be perceived that way. I understand the law, I support what the law makes available, but I do not trust the government and establishment to be fair.

We know of the syphilis experiment and Henrietta Lacks and how oftentimes we have been used as human guinea pigs. If I had a magic wand that would ensure that no person at all, no matter who they are, would be discriminated against, would be experimented upon, and they would be treated fairly and equitably . . . There are studies that show if you have pain and you are black, versus a white person in pain, physicians think differently about whether or not you are telling the truth. And there are a lot of things to be unraveled in the history of African ancestry, people of African ancestry and their bodies in America, that I have a pastoral concern and a political concern about. If I knew that the person trusted his or her physician and had a clear personal relationship with that physician and knew beyond a shadow of a doubt as much as we can know, that that physician cared, loved the person as an individual, and that he or she would be treated fairly and honorably, and if this was that person's decision, then I would support it.

D: So what you're saying, or suggesting, is that overall, there is mistrust on the part of the African American community, or among the people you know?

REV. L: Yes.

D: About whether physicians would be acting honorably, or whether there might be some underlying racist reason to suggest that life should be helped to come to an end?

REV. L: I think it moves beyond the realm of a conspiracy theory, because there's documented proof of medical malfeasance, even diabolical medical practice. A lot of the innovations in gynecological care took place because women of African descent were experimented upon. What I never want to do is lose that historical perspective. You've got the Voting Rights Act, and then in 2013, it's gutted by the Supreme Court. There are always people working on reversing justice, and returning to the status quo, for their own benefit.

D: Here in D.C., of course, we now have the right to medical aid in dying. Has anyone in your own faith community here at the AME church chosen to use that?

REV. L: No, not to my knowledge. But I feel as equipped as one can feel that if someone comes to me, we can have a robust conversation. I think about my own death. We live in a culture that seems to hide from mortality.

D: They pretend it's not going to happen?

REV. L: Yes. And you know what's fascinating in our world? Ash Wednesday. From dust you are made, to dust you shall return. I've spoken with a lot of parents, and people are concerned about being a burden to family. People are concerned about the economic realities of longevity for the sake of longevity, absent quality of life. And it seems to me to be one of the topics where truth is not found in generalization but in granularity, one conversation, one human being at a time.

D: So do you believe the concerns of the African American community are different from those of the white community?

REV. L: I think so. I think it's as real as the fact that if you are white parents, you don't have to have a conversation with your son about driving or walking down the street. I think there are things that persons of African descent in America have to worry about and think about that white people don't necessarily have to worry about or think about, because of stereotypes, because of socioeconomic and political structures. So that would be where I start the conversation. I need guarantees that people will be treated fairly, equitably, and humanely regardless of how they look, or what their cultural or linguistic or racial backgrounds might be.

D: What about the disabled community? Do you think there's a lot of hesitation there for those same reasons?

REV. L: Oh, yes. And I remember radio programs about eugenics. Let's be very clear about movements in this nation and around the world where "undesirables" were killed, were exterminated, were experimented upon. I think all these conversations must begin with robust historical contexts if people are serious about this being an equitable opportunity for persons across the board. Diane, I become very, very suspicious. For example, if you talk about Iranian American relations and you begin in 1979, I'm dubious if you don't talk about what happened in 1953, and what happened with the British when they were trying to get hold of the oil.

D: Oregon has had twenty years of experience with medical aid in dying. There has not been one question raised about treatment of any individual who has chosen to use it. In fact, of those who've received the medications over these twenty years, one-third have not used them. They've asked for, been given, gone through all the process involved to acquire the medication, but in the end, chose not to use it. But there has not been a single issue raised about anyone who's used it, no forcing, no complaints from relatives, no charges of wanting the inheritance of someone else, not one issue raised. I wonder if that gives you a tiny bit of assurance about what's happening.

REV. L: I think that is very reassuring. I think it speaks to the medical establishment that they take it very seriously. I think also, if you consider states, at least from my vantage point, Oregon's politics resonate more with an equitable understanding of how resources are to be shared and used. So that makes sense. It does give me hope. And I think that if there are more states, more jurisdictions, who can show that this is done well, I think more people of African descent in America might be willing to participate. If we're honest, people of African descent in America have decided for years to die rather than to subject themselves to certain kinds of living. During the transport from Africa to the Americas, persons would throw themselves overboard. It's even enshrined in music that we sing:

"Before I be a slave, I be buried in my grave."

D: So, the issue of trust is central to your thinking?

REV. L: If there were a group of physicians that I trusted, that I knew were respecting me . . . Let's make the assumption that the persons who would be seeking this assistance would be elderly black people. Well, I have an example of the way elderly black people are disrespected in this culture. The president of my own university got sick and he was sent to, like, an indigent space until someone saw him and said, "Wait a minute, that's so-and-so." So then he was sent elsewhere. And the reason he was sent to that place is because he was black. They didn't ask him what degrees he had.

D: Which university?

REV. L: Florida A&M University, my beloved alma mater. And there are multiple stories of people in this church who are prominent. Some of them are internationally prominent. And the way they have been treated, until someone says, "Oh, but that's so-and-so" — well, I shouldn't have to be so-and-so to be treated like a human being. I feel like it would be dereliction of duty to pretend that right will be done because it's right. It would be my fondest hope and wish, but unfortunately, it's not so often the case.

D: For you, Reverend Lamar, what would be a good death?

REV. L: A good death for me, Diane, would be to be surrounded by those I love, to feel like, hopefully, prayerfully, that I had fulfilled much of my purpose for being alive and to be able, as much as possible, to make decisions that resonate with who I am at the time of death. I would hope that someone would be able to ask me and I would be able to respond, do I want this intervention, do I not want this intervention, am I ready to cross over, am I ready to travel to the realm of the ancestors. I would hope I would be cogent enough or cognizant enough to make those decisions for myself. That would be a good death.

To quote John Wesley, who said on his deathbed, "The best of all is God is with us." For me to feel in that decision that I am tracking with the one who I feel gives life and makes life possible. I think in that way I could say, as our ancestors said, "I want to die easy when I die." I love that. There's a song, "I want to die easy when I die, shout salvation as I fly, I want to die easy when I die." And I think an easy, beautiful death, not assaulted by pain, is one of the great gifts of being mortal. I hope I have that gift.

DR. ROGER KLIGLER
A SUPPORTER OF MEDICAL AID IN DYING

Roger Kligler is a Georgetown University–trained physician and an ardent supporter of medical aid in dying. He's married, with three children. I talked with Roger in January 2018.

After undergoing six biopsies at age fifty, he learned he had prostate cancer. As a physician, he knew that even given the diagnosis he could possibly live for fifteen more years. He told himself that prostate cancer is usually a curable disease — most men who have it die of something else. But he also knew from treating his own patients that the disease is more aggressive the younger you are.

After researching all the options and listening to all the specialists, he decided to follow the course that would give him the best chance as a fifty-year-old of a cure. He opted for a radical prostatectomy, waiting through the winter season for warm weather so that he could take leisurely walks after the surgery. His wife agreed with his decision, even though, like him, she was aware that removal of the prostate often causes impotence and may cause incontinence.

Ten years earlier, Roger and his wife had seen six family members die within eighteen months of one another, his mother and his father-in-law both dying very painful deaths. At that point, he says, he vowed, "I'm not going to die that way. I'm a physician. If the time comes, I'll know what to do to take care of myself so I don't have to go through that kind of suffering."

Later, he said, he realized how unfair this was. If a death without suffering was what he wanted, and it was readily available to him, why should it not be available to others as well? He called this "the definition of justice," that what's available to one person is available to everyone in like circumstances. People who do not wish to endure suffering should have that option.

"People are not dying well," he went on. "Twenty-five percent of people who die with chronic illness die with uncontrollable pain, and that's despite hospice and palliative care. Twenty percent of people die with uncontrolled shortness of breath. At a certain point you realize, I'm not going to get better. Today is the best day of the rest of my life. I'm not going to be able to have joy in my life. I'm in chronic pain, I don't feel well, I have no energy, it's an effort to feed myself. I watched my mother die of pancreatic cancer. She'd eat a meal and then go lie down. It wasn't a life for her. She was a phenomenally bright woman who broke through glass ceilings, but now she wasn't able to live her life, she wasn't able to do what was important to her. She had a very painful death."

DIANE: But, surely the doctors caring for her must have been able to provide her with painkilling medications. Were they afraid that giving her too much medication would harm her?

DR. KLIGLER: What is harm, and who gets to define harm? My feeling is that it's the individual who should define what's harm for him or her. If I keep people alive so that they're suffering, is that doing no harm? If someone wants to end his suffering, I don't feel I'm doing any harm, and I have no ethical problem.

I've helped people die in many ways. I've had patients who said, "I don't want to stay on a ventilator the rest of my life." So we'd talk about it and I'd say, "We'll put you on a ventilator and try to get you better within a given time frame, but if you're not getting better, what do you want me to do? If I take you off, you're likely going to die." In some cases, I've literally pulled the tube out of patients and have helped them die because they've said they don't want to remain on a ventilator for the rest of their lives. Same with dialysis. Some people say they've had it, and don't want to have dialysis anymore. They've had enough.

D: What about VSED (voluntary stopping of eating and drinking), which my husband of fifty-four years had to do to end his life because medical aid in dying was not available to him?

DR. K: Well, for some people VSED can be not that painful. But for others, it can be a horror show.

D: Should family members have a say? Who makes the decision if there's no agreement?

DR. K: I believe in patient autonomy. The patient is the boss of his or her own decision making, and that's the way it works most of the time. Occasionally the family will come up with something that would supersede patient autonomy, but that is very, very unusual. Patients have the right to be able to do what they want for themselves, unless they're not mentally competent.

D: But what if a family member or a friend opposes medical aid in dying? You believe in patient autonomy, but there can be great discord in that family when the time comes.

DR. K: First of all, I am in Massachusetts, where medical aid in dying is not legal. So I could never apply it here in this state. When I had a patient ask me about giving medical aid in dying, I did not give it to him. I was a coward. I'm ashamed that I did not. I did not give him a prescription for sleeping pills so he could go home and take them and die peacefully because I was concerned that it violated the laws and that I could lose my license or, worse still, go to jail. Even if I had wanted to try medical aid in dying based upon the Oregon laws, I couldn't have done so because he wouldn't have met the law's criteria.

In 2012, an initiative was introduced to

bring right to die laws to Massachusetts. Though he didn't work on the campaign, Roger thought it was a "slam dunk" since polls had shown that 60 percent of the people were in favor. In the end, support went down from 51 to 49 percent, and the initiative was defeated after the "no" camp raised $5 million and aired disinformation advertisements on television. Roger believes the opposition came pre-dominantly from the Roman Catholic Church.

As for doctors, in a poll of the Massachusetts Medical Society taken in 2017, two-thirds of the doctors who responded felt that medical aid in dying should be permitted in the state. In December of the same year, Mass Medical changed its stance, in support of "engaged neutrality," meaning that the organization will help doctors to do things properly when they become legal.

I asked Roger about charges that medical aid in dying is actually suicide.

DR. K: The people who are dying do not want to die. I don't want to die. I'm not even sure I'd use medical aid in dying. If I do, it's not because I want to die. I enjoy my life. I love my life. I'm not looking for a quick exit. I will live as long as I can. One out of three people in Oregon who end up getting prescriptions for medical aid in dying don't take it. If you look at the statistics, one in four people end up dying with uncontrollable pain. If you wait until you're at that point, most people who try to get end-of-life medications aren't able to. They die while they're in the process.

D: What about those who live in states where medical aid in dying is not permitted?

DR. K: They're forced to pick up and move their entire households to another state. For example, Brittany Maynard moved from California to Oregon, because she had inoperable brain cancer and knew she would die in excruciating pain if she didn't have medical aid in dying. But most people can't afford to leave a job, their support structure, family, friends, clergy. And then you have to find physicians. Many doctors don't want to help people with medical aid in dying, so it's not like you can just make an appointment with any doctor. You have to find one who is supportive. And then you have to find a second one! So it's very difficult. And it takes a long time. You end up saying, "I'm going to leave my beautiful home, the things that make me feel good about life, my friends, all this when I'm going through emotional angst, and go somewhere else where I don't know anyone." It's very difficult. In some ways, it can be inhumane.

I asked about the position of the American Medical Association on medical aid in dying.

DR. K: The AMA is still debating what to do. They realize that medical aid in dying is unpopular with a large number of doctors, and they're trying to figure out the ethical position. Based on polling, it's about two to one in favor. But the AMA is never going to resolve the ethical issues because there are two ethical goods going against each other. You've got the ethic of autonomy going against the ethic of maintaining life. We're taught as physicians how to maintain life, how to help people, and we're not really taught about end-of-life care. I'd like to see that being taught in medical schools and in residencies. Nothing I say is meant to diminish palliative care and hospice, which are really wonderful, but they're not always completely successful, and you need another option.

Death is not an enemy, death is inevitable, and to be afraid of what's inevitable will blind you from living the life you should be living. And physicians need to realize this. When I was still working with patients, I would tell them that my goal was not to keep them living forever, but to try to keep them as healthy as possible. If they said, "I don't care what's going on, I want you to keep me alive as long as possible," then I would follow through.

My wife and I talk about death all the time. We even laugh and joke about it all the time, and where I'll be buried. I was speaking on public television the other day, and I tried to make a joke about death and it didn't go over very well.

I asked Roger about the difference between a terminal illness and being terminally ill. He said that having a terminal illness means you have an illness that, if untreated, will cause you to die at some point in time, whereas being terminally ill refers to having a life expectancy of six months or fewer. He describes himself as having a terminal illness.

DR. K: You're not worried about things you can't control. So now I'm sixty-six and feel as though I'm having this wonderful experience of living a second life. I call it my gift of cancer, that I've been able to go past the fact that I'm going to die, and to appreciate my life much more. If I die after all my years, that's not a tragedy. The world isn't made for us to be here in it. The world will go on without us, and we need to accept that. Once you accept that, life becomes much more beautiful.

Stella Dawson-Klein

WIDOW OF MARY KLEIN

Stella Dawson met her wife, Mary Klein, in 1980 in England, through a feminist newspaper that Mary had worked on and Stella distributed. Stella then moved to Washington, D.C., to help work on the newspaper, and she and Mary ended up living in the same group home there. They were married for thirty-seven years until Mary's death.

Their home in Northwest Washington, D.C., is quite near the house where I grew up, on a street of row houses with front porches like my own. Stella is tall and very slender, with short graying hair, and beautiful pale blue eyes that fill with tears as she talks about Mary, their relationship, their marriage, Mary's illness, and her struggle to find a doctor willing to help her to die.

STELLA: I'll always remember Mary walking in the door. She had that very distinctive sort of pageboy haircut. She was with her dog. She always, always had a dog. So she walks in with the dog, this fabulous haircut, a ribbed jacket, and a tent and a fishing pole.

I thought, Oh, this looks like an interesting woman. And I knew she was a fabulous journalist. Within three months, we'd moved into our own apartment together. When we did, I thought, This was a little rushed, and Mary said to me, "Well, Stella, we'll move in for a week, for a month. And then we'll assess. And if one of us wants to move out, we'll toss a coin." A month later, we never even discussed it and we never tossed the coin and we were together thirty-seven years.

I ask her about Mary's professional life.

STELLA: Every ten or fifteen years, Mary did something different. She was a journalist for many years. You'll have to give me the tissues — the tears are coming sooner than I expected.

DIANE: Totally understandable.

S: Yes, she was a journalist and worked for the *Cape Cod Times* and then *The Fairfax Journal.* And then she worked as the managing editor at Capital

Publications covering Great Society programs on Capitol Hill, which were then dismantled during the Reagan era. During that time in the eighties, she started getting more and more involved in her artwork. She decided to apply to art school, and being Mary, she did everything 150 percent. She was accepted into Virginia Commonwealth University, but she wanted to go to the Art Institute of Chicago. And I said, "But you don't even have an undergraduate degree in art." And she said, "I'm going to apply." So she submitted her portfolio and she was accepted.

We moved to Chicago, and she worked as an artist for the next twenty years and also did journalism on the side. She did most of her work in exploring language and how it defines and creates identities and how it's used to marginalize people. Very central to her work is her exploration of lesbian identity.

D: And during this time, you continued working as a journalist?

S: I began in radio, then did a bit of TV, and then moved into newspapers and became a journalist for Reuters. I'm now head of communications at a trust fund that's based at the World Bank. Please, give me another tissue.

D: Tell me about the first signs of Mary's illness.

S: Mary had been preparing a dog for a dog trial — dog training was her retirement job. When we were in Germany, she learned about the sport *Schutzhund,* which is for German shepherds primarily. The sport requires a very high level of obedience, agility, tracking, and very stylized protection work, pretty intensive. So she'd gone to Minnesota to train with a German trainer out there.

She'd been there for maybe a month and then drove to upstate New York for the trial. And she called me — this was in July 2014 — and she said, "Stella, I'm really, really tired." And I said, "Well, I'm not surprised, you've been away for a month and you've had a lot of driving." And she said, "I'm not sure whether I want to do this trial." And I said, "Why don't you just give it a go? It'd be a shame after all the work you've done." So she did the trial, and she said she had no energy, no interest.

This was completely unlike her. And then Mary began complaining of stomach pains and digestive problems. We put it down, again, to the fact that she'd been traveling so much, not eating well, and had always had problems with indigestion and constipation. So we didn't think too much of it. When she started having more pain she went to the doctor. She thought she had diverticulitis, which she'd had before. The doctor gave her medication, which didn't cure the problem. She went back and the doctor basically said it was psychosomatic, and Mary was furious. And she said, "I'm going to get an X-ray, this is ridiculous."

So she went and got an X-ray, and that afternoon the doctor who was reading the X-ray left a phone message for her and said to call immediately. And Mary called him back, and he said to go to a gynecological oncologist right away. When I came back from work, Mary took my hand and took me into the living room, and we sat down and she said, "Stella, I think I have cancer." And I was very British about it. I said, "Oh, don't worry, you had one tumor removed, you have

143

another ovarian tumor. It'll be okay."
And she took my hands and she said,
"Stella, I know this one's serious."

We spent the weekend researching
doctors and made an appointment,
and sure enough, it was advanced
ovarian cancer.

D: Did she go back and read the riot act
to the first two doctors?

S: Oh, yeah. But you know, the awful
thing is that her abdomen was quite
swollen, and she kept saying, "I've got
to do more exercise, I'm getting so out
of shape."

D: So, what was done for her after that
diagnosis?

S: I think we saw the doctor on a Monday, and he said he would get her in
for surgery the following week. On
Columbus Day 2014, she had about a
six-hour surgery; the cancer was quite
extensive. They removed the uterus
and ovaries and part of her colon and
part of the peritoneum. She liked to
say they stitched her back together
with forty-two industrial-size staples.
She spent two weeks in the hospital
recovering.

In November, she began chemotherapy, what they called "high-dose che-

motherapy" because with ovarian cancer there's no cure. The best hope is to knock it down the first time, and the longer you can keep it in remission the first time, the better your chances. They gave her very high doses of chemotherapy in hopes of killing the rest of the cancer cells. With that particular kind of cancer, it's not like having one tumor — the cells spread when you cut it out; they just travel, so it goes to all other parts of the body. So she went through intensive chemo, and it gave her six months before the cancer returned.

Chemo is terrible, absolutely terrible. The basic thesis of it is to kill off as many cells as you can and then let them regrow, and hope they regrow as noncancerous. The chemo was so terrible. She had multiple blood transfusions, she had blocked bowels twice, she had to have her stomach pumped. They didn't think she would survive.

D: Did Mary ever say, "Enough! I don't want it anymore!"

S: Not at that point. When she was diagnosed, Mary didn't want treatment because she knew her condition was fatal. And the doctor said, "Now is not the time to give up. I can give you quality of life." Quality of life was the driving factor for Mary, right from the very beginning.

D: Of course, quality of life in the eyes of the doctor and in the eyes of the patient are two very different things.

S: Yeah, but if she could do chemo and know there might be a week out of the month when she felt good or if, at the end of the chemo treatments, she might get three or four months when she could enjoy life, she would do it. And she did. She did five series of chemo because she wanted to live and she wanted the opportunity to enjoy her life. She did all she could for as long as she could. Then she tried "salvage therapies," which essentially means the doctors try anything that might work.

And each of those salvage therapies is more severe than the last. That's the dogs, in terms of side effects. So after the first two, nothing was working and Mary said, "No more." She said, "My body is too debilitated. No more."

D: Was that the first time you talked about the possibility of medical aid in dying?

S: We talked about it from the very beginning. From the very first day. At the time, there was no D.C. law. When Mary was diagnosed, she said to me that she didn't want to go through unnecessary suffering and wanted to have medical aid to end her life. It didn't surprise me, because Mary was very strong, very independent. And very emotionally clear. Right from the very beginning, she said she wanted access to medication.

D: And how did you feel about that?

S: I respected it. I was not surprised, because I knew her. And I knew that agency over her own life, her actions, was core to who Mary was. So I wasn't surprised, and I supported it, not because I wanted her to die but because it was cancer. That was in 2014. We looked into moving to Vermont. And Mary registered for Dignitas, the clinic in Switzerland. She signed up for Exit International, which provides information on how to take your life.

Two places where you could potentially get the medication were Mexico and Peru. I looked it up on the map of Mexico City, and it appeared to be a veterinarian you went to. I'm thinking,

This is not very good. I think the likelihood would have been that she would have decided to go to Switzerland.

D: How did your effort begin in D.C.?

S: Mary had been in contact with Compassion & Choices, and in August 2016, there was a call to action, to write to your council members and lobby, because there was a good chance they would vote on a right to die law. So we both hit the telephones, started writing letters, and Councilwoman Mary Cheh was the first person who responded. Then Council Member David Grosso got back to us as well and said he would meet with Mary. He was very concerned about people with disabilities and the argument that the law could be used by family members who wanted to get rid of them. Mary spoke very eloquently about the fact that you have to take the medication yourself, that you have to be of sound mind in order to be able to get it, and anyone who is not able to make those decisions cannot access the medication. We talked to anyone who would listen. This was in October 2016. They voted to approve in November. And the mayor signed the law in December

2016. Then, of course, Congress tried to overturn it. Fortunately, that didn't happen.

D: But you and Mary still had a difficult time finding a doctor?

S: Mary asked both her oncologist and gynecologist to write the prescription for the medication to end her life. But neither would. Right from the very beginning, she had said, "I will do everything I can to live if I can have a decent quality of life. But when the time comes when you can't do anything more, I need your help."

D: And they both reneged?

S: Yes.

D: Mary must have been furious.

S: Yes. She started setting up appointments with medical ethicists at various hospitals to get the doctors and hospitals on board with the understanding that medical aid in dying is an option they should offer to their patients. A lot of the problem was not only that they weren't *willing* to do it, they were just plain *ignorant*. All of their training was to cure. All the impetus was to give the patient more drugs, because there is an infinitesimal chance that they will live an extra month. And Mary realized it was an educational process, and that became her next task, after getting the legislation through — she now had to educate the medical profession.

After a series of meetings with doctors at Sibley Hospital, Washington Hospital Center, and George Washington University Medical Center, Mary was referred to a doctor who'd been using herbal treatments for cancer, including medical marijuana. This doctor told her that if another doctor would take the lead, he would be willing to work with her. So, after a four-year journey, Mary finally knew she could access the medication. She would be able to choose how she died, and she would be able to die at home.

Mary and Stella met with the second doctor soon afterward and really liked her. She was well informed about the legislation in D.C., having educated herself about it, and knew doctors in Vermont and Oregon. She told them that she'd never done this before, but if they were willing to go on the journey with her, she would be willing to go on it with them. She was the first person, said Stella, who connected with them as a caring physician and a human being.

The next step was for the doctor and

Mary to register. Several friends signed forms to say that Mary was doing this voluntarily and that she was of sound mind. The next challenge was to find a pharmacy. Fortunately, the doctor had worked for many years with AIDS patients and knew the pharmacists who could provide the drugs. The doctor gave Mary the prescription for the medication (which costs thousands of dollars). She got the prescription at the beginning of May, and by the beginning of July, the cancer had advanced considerably. She became increasingly tired and was experiencing more and more pain.

I asked Stella how Mary felt about palliative sedation.

S: Mary saw it as part of a continuum of care. She was enrolled in hospice and very pleased with the care she received. She didn't want to be in a coma at the end of her life. She wanted to be present, she wanted to be with me and the dogs. She wanted to be able to say goodbye. On her last day, she was having increasing difficulty controlling the pain. The doctor came in the evening, and she said to Mary, "I can give you medication so you're not in pain." Mary said she was already sleeping too much, because by then she was on a fentanyl patch and hydromorphine. She said to the doctor, "If you give me something, I'm just going to sleep, aren't I, I'm going to be unconscious." The doctor said yes. And Mary said, "No. I don't want that. That's not how I want to leave this world."

Mary had a draining tube inserted into her abdomen to take the fluid out because her abdomen had become very swollen. It was like she was pregnant. It had worked for two or three weeks but had stopped working. We went into the hospital to have it checked, and they did a scan, thinking there was just some blockage and that they'd put in another tube. But the doctor came out and said, "There's no fluid." I looked at him and said, "You mean it's a tumor," and he said, "It's all tumor now, pressing on other organs." When that happened, we knew she had very little time, that there was very little left to do. Mary said, "I think you should call everyone and tell them to come."

D: Did you know that it was going to be the end?

S: No. I still thought she had several

weeks. We had friends over and her son, and lots of people came by to visit. That was on a Thursday. On Sunday she got up early and then went back to bed. That was the last time she came downstairs. My sister and brother flew in from France and England, so she got to visit with them for a short time, and she was laughing and joking. It was really rather lovely. By then, we were both pretty tired and went to bed. She needed more pain medication, so I helped her use the bathroom and take pain meds. We got a little bit more sleep and then she woke up again, and I thought she just needed more medication. But then she said, "You know, Stella, it's time."

D: Where was the medication kept?

S: When Mary had got it, she put it in a cabinet in her workroom — her studio. I didn't want anything to do with it. I didn't want to look at it. I didn't want to know where it was. But that evening, I must have sensed the time was very near. And I asked if we could look at the medication together. The medication is an antinausea pill, initially. Then you wait an hour for it to take effect. Then there are pills, which, fortunately, the pharmacy had provided in powder form, so all she needed to do was to mix it with water and drink it. And it was instant. She lay back down and went into a very deep sleep. It was instant.

D: And you were right there with her?

S: She died in my arms. It was about two and a half hours before she passed away. It's what she wanted. It's exactly what she fought so very, very hard for. And it was very peaceful, very calm. I was very peaceful, at peace with it. It's harder now. But she had integrity. That's the person Mary was.

D: How are you taking care of yourself, now that Mary is gone?

S: That's the real question. I think of myself as a single mom now. It's a journey, isn't it? The first couple of months, you're a bit numb. And I clearly don't have a problem crying, so I think that's healthy. All through her sickness and all through this journey of trying to find a way for her to die peacefully, we did two things. One, we were grateful for a wonderful life, for many adventures, for allowing each other to live to the fullest, jointly and together. We focused on the fact that we had more time, and we took it day by day and enjoyed each day. We didn't think we'd have four years. You usually only live about two years with this type of cancer. Four years was a real gift. And it enabled Mary to do her campaigning. I honestly believe that she was instrumental in the passage of the legislation here in D.C. She was the one person involved for whom this was real. She had the disease and was willing to talk publicly. Mary is an extremely private person. It's not like her to speak publicly at all. She would prepare carefully and would get very nervous. It was exhausting for her, particularly as the disease progressed. But she felt it was so important that she talk about it.

D: Are you considering continuing her work in this area?

S: I've talked to *The Washington Post,* which is doing a story about her. I've offered to talk to partners or spouses who go through it. Because it is something to be there when someone dies. And yes, I will speak out and I will continue to do whatever is necessary if Congress tries again to overturn it. I will be back up there lobbying again.

Because if they overturn it in the District of Columbia, that sets a precedent for the whole country.

D: How would you define a "good death"?

S: It's a peaceful death. It's a loving death, and to be able to live to the fullest and live to the very end, to be able to live each moment. As to the reluctance of talking about death, I think there's a disjunction for so many people who say to me, "Well, if I'm really sick, I want to be able to just take a pill and die." It's not as easy as that. And especially right now, when medical aid in dying is not widely accessible. Death is part of living and it's a difficult journey, but the more we make it a part of our lives, the more joyful a journey it is.

DR. KATALIN ROTH

PROFESSOR OF MEDICINE, GEORGE WASHINGTON UNIVERSITY, AND MARY KLEIN'S END-OF-LIFE CARE DOCTOR

My visit with Dr. Katalin Roth took place in her home in suburban Maryland, where she lives with her husband. She is an extremely busy physician in her late sixties. At the time of the interview, Dr. Roth was the only physician in the District of Columbia to come forward to help an individual wishing to exercise the right to die. Mary Klein was her patient.

I began by asking Dr. Roth why physicians are so reluctant to help patients with medical aid in dying.

DR. ROTH: I do think there is support in the medical community for this. But it's hard to break with tradition. I'm not sure I'm the only person who's been willing to do it. I know I have some support from colleagues.

DIANE: What is it going to take for other doctors to come forward and be

157

willing to say, "I, too, will be willing to follow in Dr. Roth's footsteps"?

DR. R: I think for younger doctors, there's been some normalization of physician aid in dying. We have more than twenty years of experience in Oregon and maybe ten to fifteen years in the state of Washington. I think the acceptance is increasing. But people also worry about their employers, whether their institution will stand by them. Those issues have not been well addressed. It requires a lot of commitment from the physician to make that last journey with the patient, and many people hesitate before undertaking that.

I reminded her that there had been some sort of registry and that doctors had to go through a certain amount of training here in the District of Columbia. I asked whether doctors were unwilling to have their names publicly revealed.

DR. R: Well, I was hesitant as well. That registry has been removed. There is a registry like that in the state of Oregon. And possibly in the state of Washington. I think that it's now well accepted in those states. The D.C. law is extremely private. It assures the physician and the patient a lot of confidentiality. But that's at a cost. It means that a person who's seeking a doctor who could provide help may not know how to access one.

D: What could make that process easier?

DR. R: I'm not actually sure how I feel about it. I think having a registry with the Department of Health that would be fairly confidential and where people could make serious inquiries would possibly be enough to preserve the privacy of the physician. As you know, my name was mentioned in an article (about Mary Klein) in *The Washington Post.* I wondered whether that would generate any kind of negative response. And actually, it has not. I'm reassured by that, and I've told people that I would be willing to help other physicians who are trying to work with their patients. I didn't really know very much about what I was undertaking, and I looked to mentors. I think it's part of the process for physicians to mentor one another.

D: Tell me how you met Mary Klein.

DR. R: Mary Klein was interested in

medical marijuana and asked her primary-care doctor about a marijuana prescription. It's legal in the District of Columbia. Her doctor referred her to a colleague of mine who prescribes medical marijuana. I also prescribe it, but my colleague knew that I might help her with medical aid in dying. He was willing to be the second certifying physician, but he wasn't ready to come forward and start the process.

D: Had you felt this way since the D.C. law went into effect?

DR. R: Actually, I've supported medical aid in dying for a long time. A lot of people who support it spent a lot of time with dying patients during the AIDS epidemic, when people were facing terrible deaths and it was very hard to help them. So it was something that was much discussed at the time. I also teach medical ethics to medical students and staff, and have been interested in the issue for a long time.

D: How did the discussion begin between you and Mary Klein?

DR. R: She told me very straightforwardly that she supported medical aid in dying and that she knew she had a terrible illness. She had metastatic ovarian cancer and was looking for a physician to help her.

D: Did she ask you directly if you would help?

DR. R: She did. And I said I would do my best. She told me about her medical history, and it's a pretty terrible disease. I work with cancer patients all the time as a palliative physician. Her cancer was very advanced at the time. She'd gone through many cycles of chemotherapy and surgery. I actually know her gynecological oncologist, and I know that he's very capable and that she had all the treatments available. I was already very interested in the law and had spoken about it at various educational conferences. And our division at George Washington also discussed how we felt about it.

D: Did you find a fair amount of agreement among the physicians with whom you spoke, or was there a lot of pushback?

DR. R: Working with geriatric people in hospice and palliative medicine, I've seen that there's a lot of genuine disagreement. There's respect on both sides, but some people just don't feel it's an appropriate thing for a doctor

161

to do. There's a prohibition against hastening death, and western medicine has been opposed to it since the time of Hippocrates. In our era, that's been a real cornerstone to our medical education. I don't think doctors can just edit that stuff out.

D: Even in a case of extreme pain?

DR. R: In the palliative world, we have a lot of experience with physicians being very reluctant to adequately treat pain because they worry about hastening death. A little bit or a moderate amount of morphine might cause breathing depression or might cause the person to drift into unconsciousness, and as I say, many doctors are very opposed to that. In palliative medicine, we've had to push back against the prejudice that doing anything to relieve pain might actually hasten death.

There's something called the doctrine of double effect. The idea behind it is that if the purpose of the physician is to prescribe pain medication in order to relieve pain, if it has an exaggerated effect or an unanticipated effect of hastening death, the doctor's not blamed because the intention was simply to relieve pain, not to shorten the person's life. But this is a tension that many physicians struggle with all the time.

D: In the last thirty years, some of the balance of power between patient and doctor has shifted. And we as patients have said we have a right to ask for and state very clearly what we want. Doctors are no longer gods on pedestals. I think the Oregon law came out of the idea that patients should have a right to say, "I'm done! I really have had all I can take." So, when someone is using medication for palliative means, and a patient or a family member says it's really not helping, whose decision should it be?

DR. R: You're preaching to the converted. I've been an advocate of patient autonomy in decision making for my whole career. And I'm sure that that affects my view on physician-assisted dying. When the choices are bad and there is no hope of cure or recovery or remission, I think patients ought to be able to make that decision, to stop treatment that's not helping, to refuse more chemotherapy that causes more suffering than benefit, and to favor comfort and pain relief over prolonged suffering.

I believe physician-assisted dying is part of a continuum. In the hospice palliative-care field, there's a strong belief that good palliative medicine can almost always relieve suffering adequately. But we've all had a lot of experience that it's not 100 percent successful.

Some people have more pain than other people with the same condition. And some people prefer to remain in control for the time they have. There is an option of knocking a person out, what we call "palliative sedation," or giving enough medication — tranquilizers and pain medicines — so that a person sleeps for the rest of his or her few remaining hours or days. Some people prefer that. Some people say, "I don't want this suffering anymore, just let me sleep." And that does not mean we hasten death; we just give them more medication so that they're not conscious.

I offered that to Mary at the very end. I said, "I could give you enough medicine so that you would just sleep for the rest of the time you have." And she said, "I don't want that. I want to be in control of when I go." In physician-assisted dying, there are some people who prefer to have that control.

I asked Dr. Roth about the medications, and exactly what is prescribed.

D: Are there differences between what's prescribed in Oregon, California, and D.C., or is it all the same?

DR. R: I'm no expert. I requested advice from a doctor in Washington State when I wrote my first prescription, and Compassion & Choices has a doctors' hotline. They were very helpful. I wrote the first prescription in April 2018, and then wrote two more prescriptions for two other people, one of whom used it, and the other chose not to. It depends on availability of medication, it depends on insurance. Not every insurance company will pay the cost of the medication, and not everybody has the means to pay for it out of pocket. Secobarbital is expensive, more than $2,000, and even higher on the West Coast. There are other medications that are available, other combinations that people use. But it's very onerous to swallow all the pills. It's a lot of pills. It's not really very easy to make death happen with medication that's ingested. It's hard. And when people are very sick it's *really* hard. Mary had a bad stomach. She was no longer able to eat. And she had a bowel obstruction from the cancer all over her abdomen. I say that because it's not an easy thing to take a hundred pills or even drink a glass of water.

D: Did you visit Mary on the day she died?

DR. R: Yes, I did. I visited her four days before she died and then again on the day she died. I think it's important for you to know that I often visit patients at home. And not only people who are contemplating physician-assisted dying, but when people are very ill or homebound and can't come to us.

D: She must have been comforted by your presence.

DR. R: Well, we visit people at home, in hospice, in geriatrics. I'd like to put in a little plug about house calls. I think they're important. People are at home, and they need to be visited where they are. Mary was a terrific person, a very impressive, admirable person.

D: Were you there with her when she died?

DR. R: No, I was not. Her wife, Stella, was there. When I visited her the last time, I did go over the medications with Stella. That was actually the first time I had seen what the pharmacist had dispensed. Mary was waiting for her family to arrive from Europe. She had a very clear idea of whom she wanted to see. But she was very, very ill when I saw her the last day. Although the timing of her death was chosen by her, by her and Stella, she was very close to death that last day. When people are dying, their blood pressure goes down, sometimes their circulation is poor to their feet and their hands, their skin mottles. There are all sorts of signs of dying. And Mary was dying that last time I saw her. She died from ovarian cancer. She did not die from the potion that she drank. That just affected the time she died, but she was already dying.

I still consider myself a primary-care doctor, so I see all kinds of problems, with younger as well as older adults. I do see some patients who are nearing the end of life and who want to discuss it. It's really hard for physicians to talk about death with patients. And some people really need to talk about what's in store for them and what they're experiencing. One of the nice things about palliative medicine is that we're available for people and families to talk about what lies ahead. Death is not a taboo subject for us.

D: Do you see a change in other medical schools as well, or is it just happening at GWU?

DR. R: There's certainly a lot more being taught now than when I was in school. I think there's a movement in that direction. But physicians are highly motivated to resist death and to go on fighting disease.

D: What would you consider a good death for yourself?

DR. R: I haven't thought about it very much. I probably would like to be able to say goodbye to people. I don't think I'd want to have a big party with everybody watching, but something more private with close family. Stella got into bed with Mary, you know, and held her. I think that was just a beautiful thing that she did. And I think I would like it to be fairly private at the end, but not alone, if I could help it.

MARY CHEH

PROFESSOR OF CONSTITUTIONAL LAW
MEMBER, DISTRICT OF COLUMBIA COUNCIL

Mary Cheh is a professor of constitutional law at George Washington University. She is in her fifties, attractive, with intense blue eyes, and is the mother of two adult daughters. She was elected to the District of Columbia Council in 2006, and decided very early on that medical aid in dying was an issue she wanted to work on. She says she felt strongly about the autonomy and the ability of people to make their final choices. In 2011, she began gathering materials. It felt like the right moment to propose legislation, since marriage equality and other major social issues were also being considered at the time.

I asked her how other members of the council reacted when she first broached the issue of medical aid in dying.

MARY: The chair of the health committee, whose support would be needed

169

for the initiative, suggested it would be better to wait until some of these other social issues had worked their way through the council, because people need time to adapt to changing social circumstances, especially with big issues like this. So I agreed to wait. And it actually wasn't until 2016 that I got tired of waiting and said, "Look, I'm doing this."

The cases that reached the Supreme Court involved very serious cancers, terminal cases, people who were suffering a great deal. In fact, because it takes so long for a lawsuit to go all the way up to the Supreme Court, most of the patients had already died. The accounts of their situations and their desire to have this option available were pretty heart-wrenching.

I asked Mary whether she had talked with any of her children about her own wishes.

MARY: Well, that's a fascinating question because I have brought it up, and my younger daughter's response was that she didn't want to have to make any decisions. She didn't feel she could handle that emotionally. And my older daughter felt somewhat similarly, but she felt, Well, somebody has to be in charge here. It hasn't been an extensive discussion.

One case involved my niece. And nobody was willing to say, "It's time." When the physician said, "There's really no hope," she was still on a ventilator and other machines. So they asked me what to do. And I had a lengthy discussion with the physician. I tried to figure out whether there was any hope whatsoever, and how my niece could be most peacefully situated so that she wasn't suffering in any way. In my family, these kinds of decisions just naturally fall to me, which is why they asked me what they should do. And I had to make the decision.

DIANE: What would happen if you're not able to let your family know exactly what you want? How would they be able to know?

M: I know that's a problem. These laws we've passed, here and in other jurisdictions, require that somebody meet certain criteria: that they be terminal, that they have six months or fewer to live, which is sometimes hard to predict. Doctors are usually optimistic.

They usually think you have six months, but you probably have fewer than that. A key feature, in addition to getting physicians to assume responsibility, is that you have to be able to self-administer. Those who cannot self-administer cannot avail themselves of this law.

When we were going through the process with my niece, there was a divide in the disabled community. There were those worried that this would be a step toward euthanasia and people who were disabled would be at risk in the future. So they were opposed to it. But there were others in the disabled community who were disappointed in the legislation because they said, "What if we cannot self-administer?"

D: For example, someone with ALS?

M: Exactly right, and I said it's not a flaw in the legislation so much as it is an understanding of what we could accomplish at this time politically, and also what people would be willing to accept. Would people be willing to accept that somebody else would administer it for you? And I thought that was a bridge too far.

D: Was the D.C. law pretty much patterned after Oregon's law?

M: There are some differences. In our law, the physician is directed to recommend to patients who want to avail themselves of the law that they be in touch with next of kin, or friends, family; that they talk with somebody. In addition, they could talk with a spiritual adviser, if appropriate. Because the faith community felt that if someone is seeking consultation, there should be a recommendation that they consult a spiritual adviser. But they're not required to do that.

D: How difficult was it to get the law passed?

M: It was not easy. I mentioned that the chair of the health committee wanted me to wait because we were focusing on other things. But in fact he was supportive of medical aid in dying. By the time I moved the bill forward, he was no longer on the council. Someone else was now the chair of the health committee, and she was opposed to the bill. If a chairperson is opposed to a bill, he or she can just prevent it from moving forward, and that's the end of it. But this woman had a lot of integrity and said, "I'm opposed to this, but I do think that people should have a chance to have their say about it." She had wanted it to be a ballot initiative. She promised to bring it to a hearing and through the committee, and we had a hearing and many, many hours of testimony. There was a three-to-two vote in the committee to push it out. Ultimately, it was an eleven-to-two vote in favor by the council.

There were two other council members who had an emotional impact on the outcome. One was Council Member Kenyan McDuffie, who recounted his own father's death and his suffering. He was so moved, he had to leave the dais, because he felt that people should be able to have these choices at the end of life, but he did it in the context of seeing his own father suffer. And another member who's no longer on the council, LaRuby May, comes from a ward that's primarily African American. There was a good deal of concern, skepticism, and perhaps even suspicion on the part of African Americans about some of these medical things. As you know, we have a terrible history of taking advantage of African

Americans in the medical context.

LaRuby May and I went over to all the different wards. I spoke to people in the faith community and other groups. When we were about to vote on this, LaRuby said, "You know what, I'm satisfied that the law has these protections in it. I'm also convinced that most people would like this as a choice. They don't have to do it, but they have a choice. On top of that, since many, many of my constituents are low income, I don't want to force them to have to travel across the country to avail themselves of a choice like this. I want them to have the same choice as somebody in the wealthier parts of the district." And that was an important position to take. As you know, the vote was overwhelmingly in favor of the bill. And the mayor signed it.

There were many people who came to the hearing to testify. We had a woman, the most wonderful woman, who was herself dying of cancer, and who became sort of the public face, saying, "I would like to be able to do this. I want to have that choice."

D: You're talking about Mary Klein?

M: Exactly right. She was very, very brave. She was quite ill, too. And she would come and testify, and she would participate in these press conferences.

D: Were there any demonstrations along the way?

M: There was a lot of public activity out there. I don't want to call them "demonstrations." It was just people who wanted to say why this is important.

Now, I haven't actually finished talking about how hard it was to pass this bill. In D.C., Congress can be the local legislature, unlike in the states, which don't have to contend with Congress trying to control their local affairs. We have something called "home rule," but Congress, anytime it wants, can interfere in our own local legislation. Congress has thirty days to pick up a bill and negate it. But they have to affirmatively vote against it, both House and Senate. Usually they can't get their act together.

The second way they can act is, when we send our budget over there for their approval, they can just line-item it out. And if they had line-itemed out the relatively small amount of money the Department of Health had to spend, they could have killed it that way. There was an effort to do that, but again, it was thwarted in the Senate, with the help of our delegate to Congress, Eleanor Holmes Norton.

The third way Congress can kill legislation is if they outright pass a bill saying, "So much of this law as it exists in the District of Columbia is hereby null and void." They could do that at any time. So even while there've been some changes in Congress since the last election, we're always going to have to be vigilant to see if a bill comes forward to try to basically invalidate this law.

D: How strongly did the Roman Catholic Church work against the bill?

M: Well, they did manifest their opposition. They made it very clear that they're opposed to this, and that no facility of theirs, no hospital, no entity that they're connected with, will be authorized to participate.

D: So now, we come to the doctors. It's been more than a year since the law has been in place, and only two doctors have stepped forward to say they will participate. What do you see as the problem there, both for the doctors who don't want to be known as physicians who will work in this area and for the patients?

M: Initially, the Department of Health was going to have some sort of registry. That was off-putting to many doctors, because they didn't want to be listed on a registry. The obligation on the part of the government is to educate people. Every few months, they send out an e-mail blast to the physician community, reminding them that this is available. The numbers are low and have remained low in part because it's a new thing. But it was never the case that we were putting the burden on the government to find physicians who would participate.

What I've seen in other places is that doctors who participate are asked by their own patients, often patients they've seen for a long time, who now find they have a terminal illness, and they have six months to live, and it's going to be painful. And that person then says to the doctor, "I know I have this option and would you help me?" That's how I think this thing will develop. The doctor might not have sought it out, because they're still under an admonition in their own minds about do no harm. Even though it might be more harmful to a patient not to help in those circumstances, there's still this aura that may make some doctors uncomfortable.

There are at least five Supreme Court justices who've said that even though you can't have assisted suicide, you can have medication to deal with your pain sufficient that even if it hastens your death, you have a right to have it. We have people doing at-home hospice and they have ports in their arms, where they can self-administer their pain medication. We're becoming more aware of the need for these options, seeing as you could be hooked up to machines.

There's also a notion that you have a right to refuse unwanted medical care, even if doing it will hasten your death. If I say to my doctor, "Take all these things off of me," and the doctor says, "Well, you know you'll die within the next two days if we do that," the doctor can't insist that you suffer medical care.

D: Mary, do you believe medical aid in dying is something you would use?

M: I don't know whether I would use it, but I know I'd like to have the choice to be able to use it if I wanted to. And you know, Justice [Sandra Day] O'Connor said in the assisted suicide cases, death will be different for all of us. And it will be. It's not unique in that we're all going to die, but the exact circumstances that we're in will be unique. Some people want to stay the course, because there's some event in their lives, maybe a child getting married, or they're expecting a grand-child, and they want to try to stay alive to be able to witness that. In some cases, depending upon what their own faith is or whether they think there's something important about staying alive as long as God wills it, that kind of thing — whatever those circum-stances are, I think people should fol-low their own path, but they should still have a choice. That's the bottom line.

When I spoke before the medical society here in Washington, D.C., I was asked questions about what would be on the death certificate. What's on the death certificate is not that I ingested a certain cocktail of drugs and died from that. What's on the death certificate is the underlying disease, because we have to put our mind in the right place here. The person is on the threshold of dying. We're just choosing how, in that little window that they have left, they choose to die. But they are dying from the disease. It's not suicide in the conventional understanding of suicide.

D: Will you continue to talk with your daughters about your own wishes?

M: I have to. I suppose part of this is my own inhibitions. They know how much I love them, and they always will. I want them to have some guidance, of course, but I have been resisting doing much more, putting that emotional burden on them.

D: One of my hopes with this book is to get families like yours to talk about this very seriously.

M: I hope that works, because there's a great need for people to confront things like this. And I don't think that as yet I've confronted it fully.

ERIC LUEDTKE

DELEGATE, MARYLAND HOUSE
OF DELEGATES

Eric Luedtke is thirty-seven years old, divorced, and the father of two children. Born in the District of Columbia, he grew up and lives in the Maryland suburbs. He holds a B.A. in government and history, and a master's in education from the University of Maryland. He has taught for more than a decade in Montgomery County Public Schools and is an adjunct instructor at the University of Maryland. He has served in the Maryland House of Delegates since 2011.

We spoke in an office that he uses for meeting constituents, about halfway between his home and Washington, D.C. I asked him for an interview because he was involved in the Maryland State House debate over medical aid in dying legislation, which ultimately failed to pass by just one vote.

DIANE: Tell me a bit about your background.

DEL. LUEDTKE: I spent the first ten years of my life in Fort Washington, south of the city, and then moved to Gaithersburg, Maryland.

D: And you became a middle school teacher? For how long?

DEL. L: Eleven great years. It was the best job I've ever had.

D: Including your present job?

DEL. L: Yeah. You know, I love the work I do in the legislature, and I make a difference. But when you work with kids, particularly kids who have a lot of needs, you see the difference you make much more immediately. You see the impact you're having on their lives in a way that, as a legislator, isn't as apparent. I know I'm making a difference, but I don't *see* it as much.

D: What led you to pursue a position in the Maryland House of Delegates?

DEL. L: Partly because I was raised to believe in public service. My mother believed in giving back to her community. She came up through the women's rights movement in the sixties and seventies, worked for the American Association of University

183

Women, the League of Women Voters, and she instilled that spirit in me. When I made the decision to run for office, it grew out of my experience as a teacher. I taught in a high-needs school. I had students whose parents couldn't put enough food on the table, families who were living in homes with two or three families, because they couldn't afford anything else, parents who were working two or three jobs. And you realize pretty quickly, when you work in an environment like that, that you can be the best teacher in the world, and your kids will still need more. So I got active in advocacy to try to help provide more for the kids in the community, and when a seat opened up, I took a shot at running.

D: Tell us how you first thought about the Maryland End of Life Option Act.

DEL. L: It's always been an issue I've struggled with. I was originally opposed. The reason I was originally opposed is that I have a history in my family of mental illness. Three family members have attempted suicide.

D: Attempted?

DEL. L: Yes. None of them successfully, thank God. But because of that, I feel pretty strongly about suicide. When I was originally thinking about the bill, I was thinking about it through that lens. I was worried that it would normalize suicide, that it was a first step on a slippery slope. But my opinion has changed over time.

D.: How did it begin to change?

DEL. L: It changed with the death of my mother. She contracted esophageal cancer in 2014. I was helping out as her primary care giver, spending a lot of time with her, going to appointments, chemo, radiation, all the treatments. It was a very difficult experience. My mother was an incredibly strong woman, and when she was sick, it was the first time I ever saw her cry. As you know, esophageal cancer is a very painful disease.

She had trouble eating because it hurt to swallow, she had trouble keeping her weight up. In 2015, we briefly thought she was in remission. But they found that the cancer was still there.

D: Oh my, how old was she?

DEL. L: She was seventy when she passed, so sixty-nine through most of this.

D: Very young.

DEL. L: You know, as a child, you have this idea that your parents are going to live forever. And particularly for me, with a mother who was such an extraordinary woman and so strong, I didn't think anything could defeat her. And then in the summer of 2015, when the cancer came back, she made the decision not to pursue further treatment and passed away that August.

D: Did you accept the idea that she would not pursue further treatment?

DEL. L: I am a strong believer in people's right to make decisions for themselves. And that decision was a very sad one for me, but I've never questioned it. It was her decision to make. I knew she'd been in a lot of pain and that she was struggling, so I accepted it and was supportive. We went through the process of figuring out her will and figuring out how we were going to take care of my brother, who has a severe mental illness, and how we were going to make her comfortable during her last days.

D: Did she have palliative care?

DEL. L: She did. A little bit. I mean

there's a range of palliative care you can get for esophageal cancer. She didn't do some of the more invasive versions of it, but she had hospice, she had prescription painkillers, and you know, the doctors did their best to try to make her comfortable.

D: To what extent did they accept her decision not to have further treatment?

DEL. L: She was receiving treatment at Johns Hopkins. She had a fantastic doctor who I think wanted to pursue further treatment and tried to lay out some options for her. But when she made a decision, she made a decision, and she made that clear to everyone around her. And he accepted it, I think. She was much closer to another person who worked there, another doctor who was doing a lot more of the direct interaction with her, and that doctor was very understanding and supportive.

D: Before she died, had you heard about medical aid in dying?

DEL. L: It was an issue that had been discussed in politics. So of course I was aware of that conversation, going back to when Oregon became the first state to legalize.

D: Twenty-two years ago.

DEL. L: Right. And I recall that debate at the time. To be frank, it's not something I really thought about in the context of my mother, because at the time, I was just doing my best to try to be there for her and support her, and I knew it was not legal in Maryland.

D: Had it not come up in the House of Delegates at that time?

DEL. L: It had. It had been introduced by that time, and I had been asked to cosponsor the bill and I had not cosponsored it.

D: Why not?

DEL. L: Because, originally, I didn't support it. I had concerns that I felt justified opposing it. As an elected official, I do believe we should take strong positions on things. And we should let folks know where we stand and why. But on that issue, I was tremendously conflicted.

D: Can you tell me, if you can name them, your oppositions to medical aid in dying? I realize that you had experienced suicide attempts in your family. What was it about the bills as put forward that gave you concern?

DEL. L: My concerns at the time were

not so much about the details of the bills. They had more to do with the issue on an abstract level. I'd say the two biggest things that gave me pause were the concern about normalizing suicide; and, there are some folks in the disabilities community who feel strongly opposed to aid in dying because they believe that it could be abused. I do a lot of work with that community, so I was sympathetic to their argument as well.

D: Abused how?

DEL. L: I think there's some concern that people with disabilities might be pressured to take advantage of aid in dying. Now, under the legislation that we passed through the House of Delegates this year, I think there are enough protections to prevent that. But I heard from a lot of folks I respect in the disabilities community about their concerns.

D: The African American community also voiced strong opposition. Did you sympathize, recognize, understand their concerns?

DEL. L: Maryland is a state with a very large African American population and a very large Roman Catholic population, two communities that are relatively religious and that have expressed moral qualms about aid in dying. I have constituents that fit in both those groups, and I've heard from them. I think elected officials should pay attention to moral concerns, but, ultimately, it's not our responsibility to impose one religion's morality on everyone.

D: How did your mother's death help you change your thinking?

DEL. L: I was there, along with my ex-wife, to take care of my mother as she was dying. It was very difficult to watch. She was obviously in extreme pain, even with all the palliative care she was getting. She was also a very proud woman and didn't like the idea of me taking care of her, particularly in the sorts of intimate ways you have to when somebody is dying. A few days before she died — one of the last times she ever stood on her own — she went into the kitchen and got the bottle of liquid morphine that she'd been prescribed, and tried to drink it, tried to commit suicide. We took her to the hospital, and she had not taken enough of it to kill her. In fact, she hadn't been able to drink all of it because of her throat; with the esophageal cancer, it was painful for her to drink. And the doctor sat us down and said, "She's going to be okay, she's going to sleep for a little while. But you know she is terminal. It's within a matter of days." And then he sort of pulled us aside quietly and said, "If she does this again, don't bring her back. It's not worth putting her through that."

D: Wow.

DEL. L: And we took her home and a few days later, she passed away. She went into a coma and was in a coma for about twenty-four hours.

D: How did they have to treat her to counteract the morphine?

DEL. L: They actually didn't do much treatment there. They didn't want to do anything invasive; they didn't pump her stomach or anything like that. They just let the morphine take its course. She slept for twelve straight hours after that.

D: It's so interesting that she was given palliative care, but that it didn't do enough to ease the pain.

DEL. L: A person can never be inside another person's body and feel what he or she feels. My mother was on some very strong pain medication but she was still in pain, and she said as much. I think the doctors were doing the best they could to manage it, but I think it became unmanageable.

D: Did you speak with the doctors about that and whether there was more they might have been able to do?

DEL. L: I did, and they told me they had given her as much as they could give her without her going into a coma or dying from the medication. And so we left it at that.

D: So her death and the way she died began to change your thinking. Tell me about the process you went through.

DEL. L: In the immediate aftermath of her death, I was in grief, obviously, and I wasn't thinking about politics. But after a couple of months, you know, we were going back into legislative session. She passed on August 22, so in January, I began thinking about the bill, which I had refused to cosponsor in the past. And thinking about my mother and what she went through, I began to question whether I had the right, as an elected official or even as her next of kin, to make that decision for her. I think her death would have been less painful, and there would have been more closure, had that option been available to her.

D: Did she at some point ask to die?

DEL. L: She told me she wanted to die.

D: What was your response?

DEL. L: My job was to be as sympathetic as I could, and I told her that I understood and that I'd be there for her and do everything I could to help her, but she didn't directly ask for the means to die. She just stated she wanted to die, and we never really had that conversation.

D: So she was ill from the time she was first diagnosed with esophageal cancer until she died in August 2015. During that time, did you have any conversations with her about what she wanted at death?

DEL. L: We did. I was given her medical power of attorney. I was there with the doctor when she walked through what she did and did not want. She didn't want extreme measures, she didn't want to be resuscitated, and I knew all that. The conversation never reached medical aid in dying because it wasn't legal. My mother was a rule follower.

D: Did she talk about any of the states where it was legal?

DEL. L: Yeah, but in her mind, if it wasn't legal, it wasn't okay.

D: When you decided to sign on to the bill, what did opponents say to you? How did they approach you?

DEL. L: The opponents of the bill, over the course of the last couple of years, have largely focused on religious arguments, moral arguments. That's most of what I heard from people. And I respect people's opinions and listen to everyone's points of view. But as I said before, ultimately I don't think it's the government's job to impose one religious view on another group of people. I've had extensive conversations with people who are opposed, because I believe everyone should be heard out. I've shared the story of my mother with people, and I think even most opponents of aid in dying understand where I'm coming from.

D: What kinds of arguments did they use?

DEL. L: I think the one I heard most often is that life is sacred, that it's God's decision when someone dies. You hear that a lot. In the last couple of years I've heard fewer arguments about normalizing suicide. I'm not sure why that is, since it was a prominent argument in the early years of the bill. But the argument that life is sacred and God is the ultimate decision maker in terms of when people pass, that's the one I hear most often.

D: And what about from the disabled community?

DEL. L: I think that community is to some extent split. There are folks who feel pretty strongly against aid in dying, and there are a number of prominent disabilities organizations that have taken that position. But the disabilities community has a strong thread of independent decision making running through it. Historically, the discrimination against people with disabilities has centered on the assumption that people with disabilities can't make decisions for themselves. And I think there are plenty of people in the disabilities community who feel like this is a decision they should be able to make for themselves.

D: And what about from the religious community? Do you see any divisions there?

DEL. L: Yes, absolutely. You have a large cohort of people who are opposed to aid in dying for religious reasons, but then you also have folks from some faith traditions who feel that people should have the right to get aid in dying. I had a rabbi in my district e-mail me, after we voted on the bill in the House, and he said his interpretation of Jewish law is that aid in dying is not okay. Then he said, "But I don't think the House of Delegates should make law based on any one religious teaching." And he said he supported my vote. That was a pretty profound statement to me.

D: The Maryland End of Life Option Act went through a number of legislative sessions. Four or five in all. Tell me what happened in this last session.

DEL. L: For the first few years, the act wasn't brought to a vote because traditionally, if the votes aren't there in committee or on the floor, we don't bring a bill out to the floor. This year, the votes were there, and the bill came out of the Health and Government Operations Committee. We had a debate on the floor and it passed by an extremely narrow margin, but it did pass and was sent over to the Senate. And then, the Senate committee watered down the bill with amendments, to the point that it would have been very difficult for anyone to actually make use of the law.

D: What kinds of amendments?

DEL. L: Requiring people to go through a lengthier process of getting approval from doctors, reducing the protections for liability for doctors, things that would have made it very difficult for doctors to actually prescribe the medication involved in the bill. As a result of that, a number of the organizations that had been supporting the bill started to withdraw their support. But the bill was brought up for a vote on the Senate floor anyway, and it failed by one vote.

It was a very closely fought issue the entire time, in both houses. We had a very emotionally wrought debate on the bill when it came to the House floor. I spoke about my mother. One of my colleagues spoke about her experiences as a cancer survivor. It was a very difficult conversation to have. The bill went over to the Senate, and I think a lot of senators were struggling with the issue. There was an effort to whip the votes, to get the votes together to pass it. It was on a relatively short time line because the lead sponsor in the Senate was called up to military orders. So they had to call the vote before he left. But when the vote came up on the Senate floor, they had a pretty — again — emotionally wrought, tense debate. And it failed by one vote. There was one senator who did not vote at all.

D: I understood it was close to a tie, for a while.

DEL. L: It did end up one vote short of what it needed to pass, with one senator not voting. I think the advocates and the lead sponsor are now considering how to bring it back next year, and how to make sure it gets through this time.

D: And just a week after the vote, the New Jersey Legislature passed the Medical Aid in Dying Act, based on Oregon's law. How did that make you feel?

DEL. L: I was disappointed when our bill failed. Maryland tends to look at a cohort of other states that do certain types of legislation almost in tandem.

New Jersey is one of them. New York, Illinois, California, Hawaii, Washington. As more of those states have begun to legalize medical aid in dying, it becomes more likely that Maryland will. So it gives me some hope.

D: What would be a good death for you?

DEL. L: I'm going to answer in the context of my mother. I think it would have been a good death had she been in less pain, and been able to be with us to say goodbye, had there been some knowledge of when it would end. I think a good death would have been a death where she was more comfortable with the process of dying.

D: Were you with her when she was dying?

DEL. L: I was. But we didn't know when it was going to come. And she had gone into a coma. We had sort of said goodbye, but there was no moment of closure and that was difficult. Earlier today I was at the funeral for the Speaker of the House in Maryland. And the priest spoke of death and how difficult it is for us to comprehend death. He said, "You know, death has been a part of life as long as humans have been alive, and we still don't really understand it." He said that "lack of understanding leads to fear, but fear is normal." What he left unsaid, I think, is that a good death is a death where there's closure and where one can be around one's loved ones and look back on a life well lived.

I think this is a very difficult debate for a lot of people. But I think public opinion is shifting nationwide. In my legislative experience, the closest comparison is with the legalization of gay marriage. When I was first active in politics, and as an advocate in the late nineties, we didn't think that was likely to happen. Now it's legal nationwide. I think we're seeing a similar shift in public opinion with aid in dying, and I think politicians will make the right decisions as we move forward.

ALEXA FRASER
A DEATH WITH DIGNITY SUPPORTER

Alexa Fraser lives in a lovely home in Rockville, Maryland, where I spoke with her in July 2017. She greeted me warmly. In December 2016 she had been diagnosed with soft-tissue cancer of the uterus, and now her light hair was just long enough to cover her scalp, having begun to grow back after surgery and chemotherapy — her final round of chemotherapy had been in May. Alexa has a Ph.D. in environmental studies and did a lot of work on human health exposures. Then she decided she wanted a different career, so she studied to become a Unitarian Universalist minister. At the time of our conversation, she was an intern at a local congregation.

I asked Alexa to tell me about her father, a very handsome man whose portrait hangs on the wall behind where she was sitting. He had Parkinson's disease, she told me.

ALEXA: Well, my dad was a guy with a lot of flair. He started something called the Open University of Washington, which was a place people could go to take a class in something fun. Playing bridge, sailing, how to marry a millionaire — that was one of his classes — bringing people together. He actually sold the business to a friend but went on running tons of classes. My parents got divorced when I was quite young. He never married again because it was way too much fun to date as many women as he could.

DIANE: And how old was he when he was diagnosed with Parkinson's?

A: He was in his late eighties, about eighty-six. He had had essential tremor, which is a condition that causes your hands to shake. When exactly that transitioned to Parkinson's, it's hard to know. By the end, he had other symptoms, including rigidity. He was normally very athletic. He swam all his life, he ran, he loved to sail. He had such an active and full life. He wrote and directed plays that were produced off Broadway, and was involved in theater here, too. Whatever was fun, he wanted to do, and he did it. But I noticed he was shuffling rather than walking.

D: I gather he lived independently.

A: Yes. He was about three miles away, which was actually very convenient to my son's school. He picked him up several days a week at school, and they were the best of buddies.

D: How quickly did the disease progress?

A: Well, from what I could see, it was not progressing all that rapidly. But apparently he started to fall. And those falls made him very scared, because he loved living independently, and because he had, for a long time, planned to control the end of his days. Parkinson's is not, as you well know, a way that you want to end your life. He had a plan, and he knew that if he fell and broke something and ended up in a nursing home, he would not be able to implement the plan. Those falls were a ticking clock for him. In fact, the night he first attempted to end his life, he wrote me an e-mail that said, "I just had my fourteenth fall, the worst yet, love you so much." And that was it. And I thought, Oh dear, fourteenth fall doesn't sound good. He was sounding fatalistic about that fourteenth fall. It was also coming up on VE Day, and he had been a POW in Germany. So I think, being a dramatic man, he chose a day to die that was meaningful to him.

He had collected pain pills, and he took quite a lot of those and they didn't work. Then when he didn't die, he moved to Plan B, which was a box-cutting knife. But when you have a terrible tremor . . . It didn't work.

D: He thought he could cut his wrist?

A: Yes.

D: Did he tell you he was going to do that?

A: No, no, no. He did not tell me any of this beforehand. I got his e-mail and time went by. Usually we were in touch once a day, and after too much time had gone by, my husband and I went to his house — this was about thirty-six hours after I received that e-mail. He was lying on his sofa and explained what he had done with the pills and the box cutter. He actually made a joke, something like "I tried these things and who knew that they wouldn't work?"

D: So he must have had a Plan C in mind?

A: Yes. He had a gun in the house, which he'd had since I was a child. As we later discovered, that was Plan C. After helping him freshen up and having some food, we left him.

D: He asked you to leave?

A: Yes. It was about 1:00 a.m. at that point. And he said, "Good night, bye."

D: Did you have any idea what he intended to do next?

A: He didn't say anything, but there's no way he would have started down that path without intending to finish it. I can't say I'm surprised that he was successful in the end.

D: He used the gun to take his own life? That must have been awful for you.

A: It was terrible. But he had done what he wanted to do. I don't get a say about what happens. He was a resourceful man, and as I say, he knew what he wanted to do. And I support his choice. He knew what made his life worth living, and he knew what wouldn't have made his life worth living.

D: Did he ever seek help — from Compassion & Choices, for example? Did he seek help from his own doctor, or express to his doctor that he didn't want to go on living this way?

A: Not that I know of. Maybe there's something about a daughter-father relationship in terms of his protecting me a little bit from knowing where his thoughts were. I did get e-mails that said, "The just-in-case folder is in the so-and-so." But I'd gotten those all my life.

D: Had you always been an advocate for the right to choose, even before your father's death?

A: Absolutely. The General Assembly of the Unitarian Universalist Church voted to support it back in 1986. And let me be clear about that: it means a person in failing body, sound mind, making the choice. We're big on choices. So I can't remember ever having a thought that the right to choose wasn't a legitimate thing. Who needs somebody else to paternalistically say what I need to do? Now, I'm not talking about a permanent solution to a temporary problem. If somebody is depressed, he or she needs treatment. But there's no going backward on the deterioration of Parkinson's. It goes one way. I can't blame him. I can't question it.

D: You said, when you were on my program a few years ago, that the right to medical aid in dying is the next civil rights issue.

A: I think that's true. As I understand it, the origin of *not* being able to take your own life is that the king owned your labor, and if you took your life away, you were decreasing the king's wealth. Well, we don't live in a monarchy. I think the laws today are a reflection of religious beliefs. And that doesn't feel right to me. No religion should have the standing to take away choices, reasonable choices, from people who don't belong to that religion. If this law were in place in Maryland, my dad wouldn't have had to pull out a gun and shoot himself. My husband wouldn't have had to find his body the next day.

When I have testified in Maryland (on behalf of Death with Dignity), there are legislators who say we wouldn't need this law if we had free guns. And I said to one of them, "My dad almost moved in with us. That could have been my fifteen-year-old son finding his body. Don't talk to me about widely available guns being a solution to this particular problem!"

D: Did any of the legislators respond?

A: You know, certainly there are legislators who understand the value of this, and there are legislators who are doctors. And let me say, I am a tremendous supporter of hospice. I believe in the support that chaplains and palliative care can give people. I want people to get all the support they can, and then at some point, they make their choice. Maybe that day they decide to shorten their life, but that's a day they can be with their family, rather than saying, as my dad had to, "Bye guys, love you, time to go now."

D: Suppose several years down the road you find your death is likely to take place, say, within six months?

A: I'm not someone who sees value in intractable pain. That's just not who I am. If I am in intractable pain, and the doctors have done what they can do with some likelihood of success, there's that expression: Are you prolonging life or are you prolonging your death? I would definitely consider taking action. You know, my dad was very brave. Not once, not twice, but three times, he did what he could to get to where he wanted to go. I think if Maryland doesn't pass this law, if D.C. undoes this law, I think I would move to California. Ironically, that's where Brittany Maynard had to move out of. But I want my family around me, and I want it to be peaceful enough that there is something to share.

D: It would mean that you would have to leave your beautiful home, you'd have to leave the place where you and your family have been so happy for so long. What would that mean to you, if you had to move to take up residency somewhere else, just to have the kind of beautiful death you wish for?

A: I would be enraged, because who is somebody else to tell me what I can and cannot do with my own life? I strongly believe the law should make choices available. It could be that this cancer comes back and I'm gone before you know it. Or, it could go to my bones, become intractable. A long, drawn-out process is where I'm not having a quality of life.

I'll tell you another legislative comment that infuriated me. This legislator said his whatever was expected to die in six months. She entered hospice, and it lasted a very long time. He said, "I got so much out of her last days, my kids got so much, all of the family got so much. And," he said, "she lived much longer than the expected time." And I wanted to say to him, "How did you become the center of this story? How did you and your children become the center of this story of this woman's death?" Who knows what kind of pain his mother or wife or whoever it was might have been enduring as she lived?

I think he said she lived ten years, to which I wanted to say, "Was that nine years and 300 days that were fabulous? Or something else? What was fabulous?" We're not talking about something that's just bizarre and outlandish. We're talking about something 65 percent of the population supports.

D: It seems that there is a widespread fear of talking about death. Everyone wants to push it away and pretend that death is not part of life.

A: I have kind of a fun story on that. I was doing a sermon for a class on death with dignity. And I was the oldest person in the room by twenty years or more. When it came time for the critique, one of the young ones said, "Oh, I think this is very important for your generation." And I wanted to say, "You've opted out?" And the truth of the matter is that all three deaths that have received enormous attention in our society and changed the discussion — Brittany Maynard, Karen Ann Quinlan, and Terri Schiavo — all three were women in their thirties, probably very close in age to the woman who told me it was my generation's problem to think about this. It's really worth remembering that none of us gets out of here alive.

FATHER JOHN TUOHEY
A ROMAN CATHOLIC PRIEST

Father John Tuohey is the priest at St. Charles Borromeo parish in Pittsfield, Massachusetts. He flew to Washington to speak with me about medical aid in dying, or, as he terms it, "voluntary taking of life."

He is a slight man in his fifties, very soft-spoken, but firm in his Roman Catholic beliefs.

DIANE: Father Tuohey, in as clear and concise language as you can, please tell us the Roman Catholic Church's position on medical aid in dying.

FR. TUOHEY: Certainly. The Catholic religion is a religion of faith and reason, so we have two dimensions, the first of which is the faith, which would be binding on us Catholics and accessible to all Christians. Essentially, God is the Creator and we are the creatures, and we read in the scriptures — for

212

example, Isaiah — the world was created to be lived in. And in Genesis, we have dominion and we're supposed to be fruitful and multiply, which means to take care of the garden and to fill it with life. And so, from our perspective, God as Creator creates life, but does not take life, and hence we would not have the authority to voluntarily take life. Death is a natural part of life, and we should trust the God of creation. Since God does not take life, it would certainly not be in our purview as creatures to voluntarily take life.

D: So, in your mind, it is the word of the Lord that you are quoting, and ascribing your position to?

FR. T: Well, it's the word of God, but that's also where reason comes in. From our faith perspective, taking life is contrary to human nature. Human nature is inclined to progress and to live and to be social beings. Voluntary taking of life is the opposite. It withdraws me from society. I'm naturally inclined to life and to seek life and to build the quality of my life. And so taking life is seen as contrary to that which we call the natural moral law, but which is also informed by scripture.

D: If the quality of life no longer exists in the mind of the individual, then what should be the role morally, ethically, of the Church and of you as a Roman Catholic priest?

FR. T: That's a very excellent question. In the Catholic tradition, we would say that as your quality of life diminishes, your obligation to pursue and maintain life diminishes, and so we begin to wean ourselves off things that would prolong our life. When we're just maintaining life, that is, not living the fullness of life, people would be perfectly allowed to begin to wean themselves off medications. For example, they may decide ahead of time that if such and such trauma should take place, they don't want to be put on a ventilator. One Jesuit back in the fifties made the comment that he was concerned that people might think there was such a thing as a "Catholic euthanasia," precisely because, as quality of life diminishes, we're allowed to say no to medical interventions that would prolong that life. As the quality of life diminishes, people can say, "You know what, I'm not going to go there any-more."

D: But what about medical aid in dying?

FR. T: That's where we would draw the line, the voluntary taking of life. It's one thing to say that my quality of life is diminishing. It's another thing to step in and take over the process. It doesn't solve any medical problem. It doesn't treat pain. Reports and the statistics change year by year, but only about 15 percent of hospice patients who get medication report that they're still in great pain.

And really, what it addresses is an existential sense — and the studies show this as well — the fear of becoming dependent and losing one's dignity. And those issues, I think, can be addressed through interpersonal relationships. The patient doesn't need medication for them.

D: But suppose someone had reached a point where there was no hope of resuming quality of life, and that patient asked for medical aid in dying. If he or she were a parishioner of yours, what would you say to that patient?

FR. T: I have seen that. I remember one

example in particular, a woman on such a high dose of fentanyl for pain relief that she was toxic. But there is palliative sedation that's amenable.

D: Palliative sedation would mean that the individual is kept barely conscious?

FR. T: Right. Depending on the level of pain, yes. Of course, if that's the only way to treat the pain, then we would treat the pain and the person would die naturally. Because, if the person is in that much extremis, taking the barbiturates is going to be extremely difficult for them as well.

D: Of course.

FR. T: They're going to want some palliative sedation anyway. Why not just run with that? Why take that next step?

D: What is the difference, then, if you're offering that kind of extensive palliative sedation knowing that it will indeed end that person's life? You're helping that person die, aren't you?

FR. T: Yes, and that's why terminology is difficult. Aid in dying can be a good thing, as well as the kind of approach we're talking about. Unfortunately, here's where we start to get into methods of moral decision making. If you're not a casuist, you're going to look at

216

me and say, "You're just playing with words, you're splitting hairs." But if you are a casuist, you'll say, "Oh, yes, that makes perfect sense." If you're a consequentialist, you're going to say, "Well, you're going to be dead anyway; why not make it as smooth as possible?"

On that level, we really have to agree on a moral approach to how we think these things through. As a matter of public policy, we can probably find some common ground. But since there are so many different ways of approaching moral issues, and we don't agree on a single approach, our approach would be that the person is dying as an effect of treating their pain through palliative sedation, as opposed to dying because they took a barbiturate that sped up the process.

The Catholic approach is that there's a difference between doing something that directly causes a person's death, and dying as a result of something that we're doing to try to help the person.

D: Have you spoken about this issue within your own parish?

FR. T: Yes, it does come up. The chaplain at the local hospital (there's no Catholic hospital in the area) has called on several occasions, mainly about issues such as "Should we put Dad on a ventilator because his breathing is failing? Or is it okay for us to take him off? He's on a seven-day regime of antibiotics, we're on day five, and nothing's getting better, do we have to go two more days of antibiotics or can we just say, 'He's not getting better, let's stop dragging it out?' Because the antibiotics are not going to change the course . . ." These questions do come up.

D: So, you are not against the idea of passively allowing someone to die? You are opposed to the idea of actively helping an individual die?

FR. T: Yes, the only nuance I would suggest is that sometimes *passive* could mean not doing something that ought to be done. What I would be in favor of is not doing anything that would interfere with the natural course of the person's dying. If I have a major heart attack right now, you could passively say, "Oh, well," but you'd be in trouble for not trying to rescue me. Just because it's passive doesn't mean it's okay. If the person is in the natural course of dying, then interfering is not necessary and not helpful at all.

D: Several months ago, we spoke with Dan Diaz, whose wife, Brittany Maynard, moved from California to Oregon, as she tried a number of different approaches to continue to stay alive. But, in the end, she did take her own life. Dan Diaz is Roman Catholic. He told us that his research tells him that many Roman Catholics support medical aid in dying. What's your view on that?

FR. T: I'm not familiar with those statistics. I don't know what studies he's citing. Just a few years ago, aid in dying was defeated in Massachusetts. Massachusetts is a fairly Catholic state, so I don't know if those statistics are accurate.

D: The issue has come up again, of course, in Massachusetts, where I just testified a few weeks ago before a committee of the Massachusetts legislature. I don't know whether that bill is going to pass. I do know that they've tried to pass it four or five times. There seems to be greater hope this year that it will pass.

Tell us about your clinical work back

in Oregon, and how you approached end-of-life issues there, where there is a right to die law.

FR. T: As part of my job as the endowed chair on the medical faculty, I made rounds in the ICU every day, which is where a lot of the end-of-life discussions would take place, and spoke with the intensivists and the residents. But as a Catholic institution, and as a hospital, we didn't have to deal with it directly, though we would have to deal with it in our hospice.

We didn't have inpatient hospice, so it would be in people's homes, and our stance was that if you're thinking about voluntarily taking your life, we want to know about it, because perhaps there's a symptom that we can address. One thing I think we do have to accept is that aid in dying is in many respects a last resort. Taking one's own life in a case of terminal illness is not one's first choice. So, is there something that we can help them with? Because more people get the prescription than actually use it. You would rather not do it, so how can we help you not do it? That's our approach, and it's very effective. But even if you decided you wanted the prescription, we could not write the prescription. And we wouldn't go pick it up for you. If you have it in your drawer next to your bed, that's where it stays. We couldn't be there when you took the drugs — and this was always a challenge, because people felt they were abandoning their patient. But their presence would be considered assisting them, and that's really beyond our mission.

That was always a challenge: How can I say "no" to my patient? If they were not in our institution, they were certainly free to pursue that route. But we wanted to know that they were doing it, in case we could help them first. Again, it's not anyone's first choice, and most people were very open to sharing their concerns.

D: Did you ever have a situation where a patient in hospice under your care said, "I want to do this"?

FR. T: Yes. Yes. And in fact, sometimes that's the great courteousness of the patient, informing the hospice nurse; they say, "Don't come tomorrow, because I know this would make you uncomfortable. I know Providence's teachings on this, so just to give you a heads-up." It is very nice, that they would be concerned about the con-

221

science of their caregivers as well. And it never became a challenge. People didn't leave our hospice because of our beliefs, nor did we ever discharge anyone because of their beliefs.

D: I see. In the case of an individual who says, "Don't come tomorrow," would you as a Roman Catholic priest be willing to offer that person last rites?

FR. T: That is a very good question. Pretty much, the consensus is no, we couldn't, because last rites carries with it the sacrament of reconciliation. If the person is conscious, they actually go to confession, as it were. If they're unconscious, the forgiveness of sin happens as well. And you can't forgive something that hasn't happened yet. So if I knew you were going to take the medication, last rites would not be particularly meaningful because you haven't yet done anything for which you need absolution. And of course, once you take the pills, you've kind of moved beyond. So I can't absolve you from something you haven't done yet.

D: But the intention is there and the intention has been verbalized.

FR. T: If you were a Catholic and you wanted to be anointed, you could be anointed, but you wouldn't receive the last rites, because they carry the sacrament of reconciliation. You could be anointed during your illness. Last rites are the very last time you'd be anointed. So while you could have been anointed frequently during your illness, you wouldn't receive that final anointing.

D: That seems so sad, especially for one who perhaps has been a lifelong and faithful Roman Catholic.

FR. T: This sounds very unpastoral, but certainly we would say, "Trust yourself to the mercy of your God." And perhaps I could say, "I'm sorry, I can't anoint you, but we can pray together and entrust yourself to God's mercy," And that is so we don't abandon the patient.

D: In the faith practice then, if one dies without having been given last rites, what happens to the soul?

FR. T: That's entirely up to the mercy of God. Last rites is not a requirement, just as baptism's not a requirement for salvation. Whether you were anointed or not anointed, you're in the hands of God at that point, so that decision would have no impact, from our perspective. You could have a Catholic funeral as well. You would not be denied.

D: You could have a Roman Catholic funeral if you had taken the pills?

FR. T: Yes. And even, completely outside of this context, if you struggled with mental illness and you took your own life, you could still have a Catholic funeral. The Church would say that it's unfortunate that the person felt that this was his or her only option, but we trust in the mercy of God, and the person would get the rituals to which you're entitled as a Catholic.

D: For you, Father Tuohey, what would be a good death?

FR. T: For me, I think I'd like to know that it was coming. If I can get personal for a minute, a few years ago I was diagnosed with metastatic liver cancer. We were talking months to live, and obviously that was not the case, but having those few weeks of not knowing gave me a real appreciation for the preparedness of knowing what's coming. And the fear of the unknown.

I'd like to know what was coming, so I could prepare myself for it. Now, if I die in my sleep, I'm not going to argue.

But I think I would like to know in advance so that I would be prepared. There are still things I would like to do.

D: And who or what would you like to have around you?

FR. T: Oh, my family. That's one of the reasons I moved back to Massachusetts, to be close to family. That would be the most important.

D: And that is what so many people who choose medical aid in dying talk about. They say, "When I die, I'd like to have my family with me. I'd like to do it at a time when I can still speak with them, when I can express my love for them. And have them express their love for me in ways I can hear." Many would say that this is part of the justification for choosing medical aid in dying. And I gather you'd like to have the same thing?

FR. T: Absolutely. The difficulty would be that you can't always get what you want. We had some real tragic cases where people were adamant to die at home and they died in the ambulance because there was no one home to unlock the door. You can't always get what you want.

D: A number of times, you've used the word *anointed.* Explain the difference between anointing and last rites.

FR. T: Anointing is the sacrament of anointing of the sick using oils. Essentially, it's a prayer asking for the Lord's healing comfort, whether that be a miracle of a physical nature or praying for the person, the peace of the patient and their comfort, consolation. The last rites would be the anointing you receive for the last time, and it's still anointing with oils, but the prayers are formulated in such a way that we are commending you to the mercy of God.

If I were to go in the hospital for an operation, I would be anointed, asking for the Lord's grace, for my recovery, and so forth. If I were on my deathbed, the prayers would be worded differently: "We commend you to the mercy of God." It's still the anointing with oil, but the phrasing recognizes the finality, if you will, of the situation.

D: So the last rites commend you to the mercy of God, but the anointing of oil leaves out that phrase?

FR. T: Yes. I mean, you're always at the mercy of God. But commending in the sense of turning you over to God, as opposed to God's mercy, for your healing. So maybe a better word for *last rites* would be *commendation*. We commend you to the Lord as you move forth into eternal life.

The reason we wouldn't give last rites for someone who is about to voluntarily take his or her own life is that the Church teaches that it would be a sin. As I've said, I can't absolve you of a sin that you intend to commit, and that you haven't committed. Let's say you change your mind. Well, you haven't been absolved, because you didn't do it, but you can't absolve someone ahead of time. That would be like asking permission to rob a bank.

D: Right. Suppose, then, that the individual has used some form of voluntary taking of one's own life, would you come in after the fact to give that person last rites?

FR. T.: I think I would. If somebody called up and asked me to anoint, I think I would not feel comfortable refusing at the last minute. I couldn't be part of the preparation for the person's death, but if the family were to call afterward, I would not feel comfortable turning them down. And again, I would anoint with the idea of commending you to the mercy of God. If you called me after the fact, I would come.

D: And would that be a general concept or is that your personal concept?

FR. T: I am not sure that there's specific directive on that. My pastoral side would say that you don't deny someone the sacraments, irrespective of how they got there.

D: Going back to the beginning of our conversation, can you give me a really tight, concise statement of the Roman Catholic Church's position on voluntary dying?

FR. T: Sure. The Creator does not take life, so nor should the creature. And we follow the example of the God who created us.

We are creatures. We have a Creator who creates life and does not take life. Part of that created order is that there is a natural way that we die and return to our Creator. That's the way the Creator made it to be. And so as his creatures, we shouldn't take control over the process but let it unfold as nature would have it.

D: As nature or God would have it?

FR. T: Well, God created nature, so yes.

D: If an individual wishes to continue on a path toward voluntarily taking one's life and not taking medication or continuing with palliative care, I mean what is the difference between not continuing and voluntarily moving toward death?

FR. T: The difference, from the Catholic perspective, would be that one way trusts nature, that God created the world in such a way that when the body can no longer physiologically sustain itself, it passes. The other way means, before that moment has arrived, I've decided to step in and choose that moment myself. Our teaching would be that it happens naturally, and we ought not take it over.

D: Does the Church consider the patient and/or the doctor who does move in that direction toward voluntarily taking of one's life as having committed a sin?

FR. T: Yes, it would be considered a sin in the Catholic teaching, yes.

D: What kind of a sin?

FR. T: A grave sin, because it's the taking of life. The taking of life, the unjustified taking of life, is probably the worst sin that can be committed. And so it would be grave. Now, there may be a lot of circumstances around it, particularly on the patient's part, let's say if they're in extremis and so forth. So there may be a lot of contingencies for culpability, but yes, the action itself would be considered a grave sin.

D: And what about a certified physician who may help that patient? Is that person also committing a sin?

FR. T: Yes. Yes. The writing of the prescription for that purpose would be considered a sinful act.

D: Do you see any movement within the Roman Catholic Church away from that sort of thinking?

FR. T: Only in the movement away from judgmental thinking. It's one thing to say that we consider the act sinful. But the Church — which is why I mentioned that if you're a Roman Catholic and you take aid in dying, the Church would not make judgment upon you but would look beyond the action to the circumstances surrounding it, and you would get a Christian burial. So while it would still consider the act wrong, you would not be denied a right of Christian burial.

D: But what about the doctor or the nurse who might be involved?

FR. T: Well, if they're Catholic, they always have access to the sacrament of reconciliation if they see the error of their ways, to use the Church's expression. They always have the sacrament available to them.

D: Tell me about that sacrament of reconciliation. I think we all know about the sacrament of confession, but how does that differ from reconciliation?

FR. T: Oh, it doesn't. Actually, the name of the sacrament was changed in order to focus on the effect of the sacrament as opposed to the act of confessing my sins, which I do, but the whole point is to be reconciled with God and the community. Calling it the sacrament of reconciliation focuses on why I'm confessing, not just the fact that I'm confessing.

D: If a doctor or a nurse had carried out the patient's wishes and provided a prescription and was there to help, and went to reconciliation, would that person automatically receive absolution?

FR. T: Yes.

D: And then suppose that person continued in that vein?

FR. T: Well, reconciliation presumes that you are changing your ways. It's a conversion experience.

D: I see.

FR. T: If you have no intention of changing your behavior, then it nullifies the sacrament. Faith and reason are integral to Catholic teaching. We would ask ourselves if it is good for society that people can voluntarily take their lives. We know that the death penalty does not reduce crime, and we know that aid in dying does not help the medical profession because the reason people are choosing it is not pain, or dismay. It's usually because of a lack of sense of dignity. We would ask ourselves if it is good for society to just say that when you feel like you're dependent on your family, it's okay to move on. Is it really good for society to affirm that it's okay, even when you feel you're helpless? Do we want to affirm that, as a society?

It's really the ultimate act of selfishness, because the family may disagree, but the person gets to do it anyway. So we would ask whether it is a good public policy to have voluntary taking of life.

D: In the long run, what kind of effect do you believe that medical aid in dying could have on society at large?

FR. T: We did see this when I was in Oregon, talking to legislators, because it results in ill people being pitted against each other. If I have cancer and I'm dying, I can do it. But if I have ALS and I have all my faculties but I don't have motor control, I can't. Yet we're both dying. If I'm dying of dementia, I have the physical ability to take the pills, but I'm no longer competent in making those decisions. So it begins to open up the question: Well, if them, why not us, and if them, why not me? Where do you decide that the voluntary taking of life is to be stopped, and where do you put those parameters? Where do you draw the line?

D: And what about the right of the individuals to choose to say they want their lives to end?

FR. T: I think probably a missing point

is that it's not a right, it's a privilege. In some states, just like a driver's license, the state gives you the privilege of voluntarily taking your own life, because of your medical condition, and it denies that privilege to other people. All of us have the right to say, "I've had enough, no more interventions." If it were a right, then any of us could do it, all the time. And it's a privilege that a cancer patient has but that an ALS patient does not have.

D: Oregon is working on that very issue.

FR. T: Right. When I was there, we would have these discussions and I would remind them, you know, you promised the citizens of Oregon that this is as far as it would go, it would never go any further. And so they approved it. And that just speaks to my point about public policy. Now that they've done it, they want to expand it. There are broken promises to society in some of this legislation.

D: And do you feel that Oregon is now breaking promises by trying to help those who you've already said cannot help themselves?

FR. T: If you voted for it because it was restricted to patients who had decision-making capacity and who qualified for hospice, and I voted for it because of the limits to it, then yes, you've broken a promise to me because I didn't want it to go that far, and now you're saying, "We've been doing this for fifteen years, let's expand it." I think that's dangerous.

D: Dangerous how?

FR. T: Because, whom do you trust? You know, you promised to take it only so far, but how can I trust you not to expand it later? And now I can't take my vote back because if I thought it was going to include these populations, I wouldn't have voted for it in the first place. I think there's a public trust issue there.

D: Of course, the Catholic Church has been the most outspoken opponent of these laws around the country and yet, I'm so interested that even when a patient says, "Please don't come in tomorrow," that that patient who has taken his or her own life voluntarily is not denied a funeral within the Catholic Church.

FR. T: And that's how mercy triumphs over all. That's certainly Pope Francis's message, but it's scripture as well.

Mercy. In the end, mercy. And if you've done it and you were part of the community, then we put our trust in God and we'll take care of you.

D: So it would not be —

FR. T: It's a nonjudgmental opposition, maybe we can call it that. Opposed to the action without being judgmental against those who would choose it. I like that expression actually.

D: I do, too.

FR. T: We oppose the action but will not make a judgment upon the person who does it.

WILLIAM "BILL" ROBERTS

A TERMINAL CANCER PATIENT AND FRIEND OF THE AUTHOR'S

Bill Roberts was my high school sweetheart. We "went steady" in our senior year, were voted "the cutest couple in the class," and attended our senior prom together. He was president of our graduating class and earned a scholarship to American University. Bill is nearly a year older than I am, but we graduated together because he had missed a year due to spinal meningitis, a disease that nearly took his young life and left him totally deaf in one ear. He and his wife, Irene, met at American University, and have been married for sixty years.

Our conversation took place via Skype, on December 11, 2018. He looked pale, but managed to smile and even laugh through the pain he was experiencing from prostate cancer that had metastasized to the bone. Irene was at his side. She was now his primary caregiver, though in the last two weeks of February 2019, nurses were brought in round the clock. I asked Bill how he was feeling, and he said he'd just had a nice breakfast and coffee, felt "perky," and might get out for a walk. "Every day is a good day," he said.

Professionally, Bill had been program manager of advanced weapons programs (nuclear weapons) at the Rocky Flats Plant, which no longer exists. He told me, "I retired so many times, but I finally retired in 1995. They kept calling me back and I looked at the checkbook and there wasn't much money in there, so I went back. I had been a chemist originally, but they take their best technical people and make managers out of them. Sometimes that works. And I hope it worked in my case."

I asked Bill to describe when his most recent health problems began.

"Well, Diane, this condition fell on me like a load of bricks, actually. It was almost two months ago. Before that I was a young man. I was athletic. I could do almost everything. Suddenly, my back started hurting, and that put me in the hospital the first time. I spent most of September in and out of the hospital with back problems. And finally, the doctors diagnosed my case and said it was stage IV prostate cancer that had metastasized. I also had two heart attacks, and the doctors discovered I have congestive heart failure. I guess there's a bet going with the doctors as to which one will get me first, the heart failure or the cancer.

"When I got out of the hospital I thought it was over, that my days had ended. But here I am, two months down the road. I have both hospice care and palliative care, more than a reliable backup to Irene, who is my principal caretaker, but she needs time to herself. She needs rest and relaxation of her own."

Irene says that when Bill first came home he was unable to do even the smallest thing for himself, and she didn't know how she was going to manage. "It was a learning experience for both of us."

I asked Bill what his doctors had told him before he was discharged from the hospital.

"They were very honest, very up-front. They told me my time was limited. When you hear those words, it sinks in. So I go, I guess like an alcoholic, day by day. I have to make every day count. I look forward to getting up in the morning and seeing my bride, my new bride of sixty years. She has a beautiful face and a beautiful disposition, and the doctors wish me well."

Bill and Irene live in Boulder, Colorado, where medical aid in dying is permitted. I asked about Bill's conversations with his doctors on his end-of-life wishes.

"We met Dr. Laura Hughes about a month ago, and I will see her again in less than two weeks. We've gone through the routine paperwork, signing on to medical aid in dying. She was very gentle and kind with me and walked me through the process generally, the pharmaceuticals I'll use. I feel very lucky living in Colorado and having this option. When I first got out of the hospital, I was ready to end it all right then, I felt so horrible. But being helped by Irene and the hospice folks, the palliative-care folks, I feel I have a future, albeit short. Dr. Hughes held my hand and walked me through that gently. It sounds like just the thing to do when the time comes."

I asked Bill how he would know when the time has come.

"Maybe it's the pain, the pain will get so bad. Or maybe I'll become confined to a bed. I'm an active person. I don't want to be restricted so much. I've had a great life. I've had a great wife. I'm lucky to have this option, this medical aid in dying. I think of your dear husband John Rehm, who did not have this option, and others in my family who did not, and they were brave souls. They had to endure."

I asked Irene how she felt about what Bill was saying.

"Diane, I was present for all the conversations, because it's always good to have two sets of ears to hear so you can countercheck each other. But I was already a supporter of the movement, Compassion & Choices. And Bill and I have always talked about everything. We've discussed end of life because friends have died, friends have gone on. Terrible things have happened to people we've loved so much, and now it was happening to us. When you get to be in your eighties, you realize time is running out. It's part of the life process. So we'd talked extensively about the end of life and what we want. In fact, several years ago, we made the decision to donate our bodies to science."

I asked Bill whether he'd applied for the medication needed to carry through on medical aid in dying, and whether it was now in his possession.

"Yes and no. We've applied. We have one more session with the oncologist, Dr. Hughes, to finalize paperwork and the conditions of Colorado state law with regard to this. It will be in the presence of a clinical pharmacologist who will supply me with the drugs. I have to pay a fairly hefty price for the drugs. We have a situation in Colorado where there's a "shortage" of secobarbital, which is the drug that finally puts me to sleep gently. It's a matter of timing whether I can get the secobarbital or not. So no, I do not have the drugs in my possession."

It's my understanding, I said to Bill, that he would have to be able to take the medication on his own.

"Right. That's the prescribed way. I must mix the formula, I must drink it myself. There are a couple of fluids I take beforehand that are antinausea drugs. Yeah, I have to do this on my own. I have my wife there, we have a couple of friends who will sit with us, who are, for me, the extra backbone for Irene to lean on when this happens. I worry about her and what happens when I'm gone."

I asked Bill what would be a good death for him.

"Well, the betting is on at the hospital that the heart may well take me first. But I look forward to medical aid in dying. It will be a gentle, gentle easing into whatever comes next. I have no great anticipations about the next life, but I tell you what, I'll find out and try to let you know."

I told Bill that I've always thought that, when my time comes, I'd like to have my husband, my children, my dearest friends all here for a lovely dinner, lots of champagne, lots of laughter, and then quietly, with my husband, son, and daughter, go off into the bedroom and quietly go to sleep. It seems to me that would be perfect.

Bill said he hadn't ordered any champagne yet, but thinks he will. Then he said, "But be sure to invite me to your party. That sounds like fun!"

On a more serious note, I asked Bill whether he was afraid of dying.

"I was. I have been. I've had a few incidents of anxiety. They're mainly related to breathing. I have a fear of losing my breath and not being able to get oxygen into my lungs, or the lungs failing, or the heart collapsing. But to answer you honestly, quite honestly, no. I don't look forward to it, but there will come a day and I'll be ready. Irene will be there. To hold her hand means so much to me. The day won't be that far off. I don't fear it any longer."

Two months later, on February 10, 2019, I received a long e-mail from Bill indicating a deterioration in both body and spirit. In it, he wrote: "My bad days have evened out with my good, alas, so I only go out with friends on days when I'm able. Got my end-of-life drugs last week. Stashed in the pantry. Its shelf life is six months, longer than a lot of products hiding in there. So, in a nutshell: I've taken a turn southward. Without friends like you, I'd probably be long gone."

On Valentine's Day, Bill wrote: "You are here with us. I feel it. It's a strange feeling, this dying . . . confused at the moment. Getting late. Irene has just refreshed me with cold water, my drink of choice at the moment. Not able to tolerate anything else. Diane, I'm dying, just don't know when or how. I'd like to drift off, be consumed by the waves . . . Fear, dread, or pain? None of the above, just all of the above all the time. Irene, the love of my life, keeps me strong, says it's past bedtime. What will I do without her? We'll soon find out. I do love you. I do love her. See you again one of these days, I promise. Bill."

Then, on February 17, came an e-mail from Irene: "Bill is in bed and has lost a great deal of strength. He is sweet but sometimes confused. This last week has been very difficult for him. He is very proud and the loss of control is not easy. Luckily we will start with skilled nursing tomorrow. Both of us need the help."

On February 22, Irene wrote: "Bill continues soldiering on but sleeps a lot. Pain we control with meds. We have had twenty-four-hour nursing since Monday and that has been helpful. Gray and cold — we need the sun to shine."

On February 23 came this e-mail from Bill: "Haven't been out of the house all week, now with round-th to final goodbyes. So weak. God give me strength. Irene, friends e-clock care. Misery. Have the drugs, almost down, neighbors, caregivers so nice, thoughtful. I truly am the luckiest man alive, pain and everything. Stay brave yourself, carry on the fight. I love you. Bill."

It was hard to read this message without crying. I couldn't sleep that night, thinking of what Bill was going through. So, on February 25, I called his home, and he answered! Sounding very weary and having a hard time breathing, he was nevertheless able to carry on a conversation with me for about ten minutes. He was waiting for a friend to visit, the widow of a former coworker of his at Rocky Flats, who'd died of exactly the same disease Bill had. I asked whether there was a connection, and Bill responded, "Yes, exposure to plutonium." He didn't want to say more than that, but I suspect there may be some lawsuits involved.

In the end, my dear friend Bill Roberts

died without taking the medication. His wife said his breathing became more difficult, until, at 8:03 p.m. on March 11, 2019, it stopped. I shall always miss his warmth and humor, his generosity toward all his friends, and the courage he demonstrated in speaking with me so openly and honestly about the end he knew was drawing near.

DR. LONNY SHAVELSON

DIRECTOR, BAY AREA
END OF LIFE OPTIONS

Dr. Lonny Shavelson's medical practice in Berkeley, California, is devoted to aid-in-dying requests. Since California adopted its End of Life Option Act, he has helped numerous patients through the process, and has written prescriptions for those who met the criteria. We're seated in the living room of his modest house. The furniture is well worn but comfortable.

DIANE: Dr. Shavelson, how early in your life did thinking about dying appear?

DR. SHAVELSON: The question of dying started before I was born. My grandmother, who had diabetes and kidney failure and was going blind, had a very difficult death. And the family rumor was that the doctor went into her room and asked the family to leave him alone for a moment, and then when he came out, he said she had just died. I never knew how much of this is true; it was two years before I was born. The assumption on the part of my family was that he had given her an injection out of mercy, and that the reason he asked everyone to leave the room was so that he could give her a merciful death. My mother was so affected by that story that I think I started hearing it when I was two years old.

D: Was your grandmother suffering a great deal?

DR. S: She was crying out, "God save me," or "God kill me," actually. Crying out in Yiddish, "God kill me, God kill me." And then she died when she was left alone with the doctor for that moment. Everybody in the family thought that if he *had* brought about her death, it was totally appropriate.

D: When your mother began to enter middle age, she had her own medical issues, and apparently when you were fourteen, she made a request of you.

DR. S: Yes. My mother had severe Crohn's disease, a bowel inflammatory disease that is a lot more uncomfortable than you might think. She suffered significantly through the years, had major surgeries repeatedly, but was generally uncomfortable from it. When I was twelve or fourteen, she started requesting me to help her die. We did that dance until she was seventy-five, and she ended up dying a natural death, as much as there's anything called a "natural death" these days. I'm not sure anybody has a natural death anymore. She died in a hospital. But through all of this we had an understanding that at any point in time, as her suffering increased, I would help her die.

D: How did your father feel about that?

DR. S: My father pretty much ignored it, never took it seriously. My father was a guy who generally tried to avoid conflict. So his response to my mother had been "Oh, that's silly, we're not going to pay attention to that." When my father said no, my mother would turn to me, and I took her request for suicide quite seriously from the age of thirteen.

D: Do you recall the language of your conversations?

DR. S: She said, "I need to die, and I need you to help me." She even had instructions. She wanted potassium. She somehow thought that at thirteen I could start an IV and give her an overdose of potassium. I'm not sure how she came up with the overdose of potassium. But our language was: I need the potassium now.

D: And finally, she had to go into the hospital, where she died naturally. How do you think that early experience affected you?

DR. S: I think what it did was open up the thought process about suffering. That was probably one of the driving forces behind my decision to become a doctor. I think people really started talking about this around the time of Jack Kevorkian, in the early nineties. And it made me pay more attention to the bigger picture. By that time I was a doctor practicing emergency medicine. I had seen a lot of deaths, and it made me really want to explore a lot more about what helping people to die really means. It was important to understand it better and to really get into the idea of what was still then a hidden world of people asking to die because of illness and suffering; Jack Kevorkian was just the tip of what was happening.

D: In your book *A Chosen Death: The Dying Confront Assisted Suicide,* you quote Dr. Timothy Quill, who says those who've witnessed difficult deaths of patients in hospice programs are not reassured by the glib assertion that we always know how to make death tolerable. Please talk about the realities of palliative care, hospice care, and what they can and cannot do.

DR. S: I love hospice, and I say that straight out. I think what hospice does is phenomenal in guiding people toward — I hate to use the term a *good death,* because nobody knows what that means — in guiding people toward a *reasonable* death, where they're comfortable, where the amount of suffering is minimized. I think palliative and hospice care are amazing at making death easier for people.

Yet there are limits, and I think everybody has to acknowledge that everything in medicine reaches a point where it doesn't work. I think that hospice workers have had an uphill battle in terms of getting validation. Over the last fifty years, it's been amazing to watch the growth. But on the other hand, there's been this attitude, due to the need to self-advertise, that we do a really wonderful job; we've forgotten that for some patients, the suffering goes on.

For some patients, even the best hospice death is not the right death for them, because it can last too long. It may involve being in a coma for three weeks during which the family has to take care of this inert body. And that's not what they want. It may be there's more shortness of breath than they would like to tolerate. There may be more pain. Pain is almost always controllable, but not always. And then there's the question of existential angst as some people get to the end of their lives. They just don't want those last three weeks. So, as wonderful as hospice is, there are limits. I think some patients should have the right to choose, even within the realm of hospice, that they're ready to go.

D: What about palliative care?

DR. S: Palliative care has a lot of overlap with hospice care. Palliative care, essentially, is the treatment of symptoms, so that you're not treating the underlying disease, you're treating the symptoms that are caused by the disease. In palliative care, that might happen in a realm outside of hospice, such as in a hospital, where there's a palliative-care team. A little less common is at-home palliative care, which starts to overlap with hospice. For those who are ill and suffering but can't yet get hospice care, palliative care is completely appropriate. But it has the same limitations. It's wonderful, it treats pain, nausea, vomiting, angst, all of those things. But some patients still have the right to say, "Thank you for the wonderful care you've provided, but I have another choice to make and my choice is to take medicines to die."

D: How do you respond to people like Dr. Ira Byock, who say that palliative care can take care of all pain, can deal with every issue, and there's no need for medical aid in dying or hospice care?

DR. S: Ira Byock and I have had this debate going on for about twenty-five years now. When doctors say, in any field of medicine, that they can do it all, I'll always doubt them. When they say that they can take care of anybody's end-of-life situation and make it as comfortable as the patient wants, they cannot be right, because nothing is effective all the time. Sometimes hospice and palliative care cannot alleviate symptoms. I'll give you an example. Somebody who has a large mass in his mouth from a cancer, and it's about to occlude the airway and stop his breathing, his salivating, and he can't swallow — this a person whose symptoms are difficult to control, other than sedating severely and putting him into sort of a confused, sedated state. And some patients in situations like that might say, "Your palliative care is helpful, but it's not what I want to do." It's a question of freedom.

D: So you're talking about allowing the patient to define what it is that he or she is feeling in terms of pain and/or suffering?

DR. S: Correct. I think that when someone like Ira Byock says we can take care of everyone and make them comfortable, there is no such thing as "everyone." Individuals should be able to make different choices than the ones Ira Byock would like them to make. There's a certain element of paternalism that goes on here — this is the old style of doctor, right? "I'm your doctor, listen to me. I can make you do the following things and you'll be fine." There's a new way of doing medicine, which is to listen to the patient, and if the patient says, "Doctor, I know you can keep me semicomfortable for the next three weeks, but I'm going to be in a stupor and sedated from all the morphine you're giving me and all the rest. I don't want that." The patient has the right to make the decision.

D: You're talking about giving the patient more choice. You, as an individual, have come to give the patient more choice, but what kind of teaching is going on in medical schools these days? When you went through medical school, I don't think there was discussion about the patient's right to choose.

DR. S: No, I think that in medical schools today there is more information given about patient autonomy and information than there's ever been. When it comes to this very difficult question of the right to die, the right to take aid-in-dying medications, I think that specific aspect of autonomy is not taught at all, not yet. It's too new. What we see in California is that we have a new law now, almost two years old. Two years is a dot in the history of medicine. And medicine always moves at a glacial pace. It might seem we're making all these new discoveries all the time, but when there are changes in medicine, they actually happen rather slowly, especially in the adoption of new practices. When it comes to aid in dying, there's virtually no teaching about it yet. It's simply too new.

D: Even hospice does not yet accept the notion that they can help a patient die?

DR. S: The fundamental principle of hospice is that we do not hasten or delay death. That's their bible, their founding principle. In other words, they allow the so-called natural flow of death to happen, and they will be there to make you more comfortable and all that. We use morphine, we use everything else. But nonetheless, hospice will not interfere with the process of dying. When aid in dying comes along, that's obviously an interference with the process of dying in the sense that you're allowing a patient to take a medication at a certain time. Hospice care has traditionally been in conflict with this. People have been afraid of going into hospice because it's viewed as the place you go to die. But hospice workers want to have a reputation of hospice as the place where you go to get help. If they accept aid in dying, it becomes the place where you go to die.

The initial response of hospice to the aid-in-dying law was one of tremendous opposition. If our patients ask for this, we're going to tell them, "Don't worry about that, we can help you, you don't need this." But as time goes by, and as patient after patient after patient since the California law passed has been asking for aid in dying, starting with the nurses who get those requests and starting with the chaplains and social workers getting request after request from patients, the hospices have started realizing that if they want their patients to have autonomy, they have to start responding to these requests.

I can tell you that in the Bay Area, roughly 60 percent of the hospices we work with now openly work with their patients with aid in dying. You need two physicians to okay an aid-in-dying request. Many of the hospices are now responding to that, and their doctors are becoming the consulting doctors. So what we're seeing is that if you ask the National Hospice and Palliative Care Organization their position on aid in dying, you will hear the traditional no, they don't want to talk about it, they don't want to think about it. But if you look locally in my area, and at the hospices I work with, you'll hear them saying, "Sure, who's the next patient?" We're seeing a massive change, very rapidly, in the attitude of hospice.

D: What about the doctors themselves? To what extent are you seeing a growing number willing to participate with hospice if they have a patient who will die in six months and says, "Doctor, I've suffered enough"? How many doctors are willing to participate?

DR. S: This is the access question. How do patients access the aid? They have a new right to under the law. They have the right to aid in dying. They have the right to hasten their death if they want to. But they need two doctors to help them. Let's just say that access to medical care is unevenly distributed in all aspects throughout our state, in some places severely limited.

D: And throughout the country. Rich people and poor people, insured people and uninsured people.

DR. S: There is not even distribution of access to cardiac catheterization, to early mammograms, and there is the unequal access to aid in dying. That said, more doctors need to be trained. What we hear from many doctors who don't want to do it is that they're not comfortable with it. It's not that they're opposed, it's that they're uncomfortable because they don't know medication dosages, they don't know the protocols, they don't know the paperwork, they don't know how to bill it, because there are no billing codes yet.

D: So what kind of instruction process is available?

DR. S: There is no instruction process available. There are people like me and our practice, and we do hospital grand rounds and do as much as we possibly can, but there are only a few of us so far. I find that it's improving over time. There are more doctors willing to participate now than there were two years ago. But access is still very difficult, especially in the more rural and poorer areas, and especially with uninsured patients, like everything else in medicine. Will it stay that way? I don't think so. I think the teaching will start happening on a more formal level. We're working on it. I think the word is getting around as there are more patient requests. When a doctor gets one request from a patient, that doctor can say no. But with the second or third request, the doctor is thinking, I better get more comfortable with this, my patients are asking for it.

D: When a patient asks a doctor who says no, will that doctor then refer the patient to someone else who may be practiced and comfortable?

DR. S: That depends on the doctor's attitude. Some will work very hard to find someone else, and some will just tell the patient to go find someone yourself. Again, we are at an early stage, and time will tell how rapidly this is going to advance. I think it's going to move fairly quickly.

D: Isn't Oregon a sufficient example for those of you in California?

DR. S: Oregon is 10 percent of the population of California. They've been doing this for twenty years. They're mostly a rural state. They are more focused on general practice and family practice than we are in this state. It's very difficult to make Oregon to California comparisons. We picked up a lot from Oregon, their medication, Seconal, and we picked up some of their styles of practice. But now our medicines have changed, our styles of talking have changed.

D: With changes at the grassroots level, before things get to the university level of teaching doctors how to speak with patients who are ready to die, it's working its way up, instead of coming from the top down?

DR. S: You're so right that it's grass roots. The demand and the need and the education are being driven by patients. Interestingly, it's driven from patients to nurses first, because nurses are the ones working most closely with patients, especially in hospice. The real power is coming from patient requests. We've had in our small practice more than six hundred requests for help with aid in dying, not necessarily all valid, not necessarily that we accept them all, but six hundred people nonetheless.

The best story I have about how this is grass-roots–driven comes from working with a patient when I first started doing this, a ninety-six-year-old woman whose heart was failing, who was in hospice. But that particular hospice did not approve of aid in dying. In fact, they referred the patient to me, and they told the hospice staff they could not be there on the day the patient died. So I went to the patient's home on the day of her aid in dying. And at the home were the hospice nurse, social worker, and chaplain. And I said, "What are you guys doing here?" And they said, "We're not about to abandon our patient." So when I say that it was patient-driven, this is exactly what I mean.

D: What a wonderful story! Now, did that patient meet all the criteria of the California law? Had two doctors determined that she would be dead within six months? How could they know?

DR. S: Everybody acknowledges that the ability to make an accurate six-month prognosis is pretty lacking. We have a hard time zeroing in on that. And I'll tell you why it's not really as relevant as everybody thinks. It's not like you

262

come to me and I tell you, "You know what? You have breast cancer, and you have less than six months to live," and you decide right then to take aid-in-dying medications. What happens is that you wait to see how sick you get. We don't see people newly diagnosed who ask for aid in dying, and we don't see people newly prognosed who ask for aid in dying. They get sick, they watch what's happening, and by the time they're asking for aid in dying, their prognosis is really evident. They're close to death. If I'm not sure of a prognosis, I tell the patient very directly.

D: So, do you believe the six-month prognosis is one of the difficulties with the California law?

DR. S: No. Given the fact that it's difficult to make a six-month prognosis, I don't think that really changes how well we function with this law, nor does that mean it's a good or bad law. I think it's important that we have some parameter to determine who qualifies and who doesn't, so that we distinguish — and this is very important — aid in dying from suicide. Aid in dying is for people who don't have the choice to live. This is why it's not suicide. People who are going to commit suicide have the choice to live and choose to end their lives. People who are doing aid in dying don't have the choice to live. They're choosing the way they will die. That's why we don't use the term *physician-assisted suicide* anymore. That's why the law says we can't write *suicide* on the death certificate even if we wanted to, because this is not suicide.

D: Let me ask you about the fifteen-day waiting period for patients after they've been given that six-month prognosis. That fifteen days might feel like an eternity to a patient who is ready to end it all.

DR. S: The fifteen-day waiting period is probably the most ill thought out and onerous part of this law. It is completely incorrect, for a variety of reasons. I think it was initiated to make sure that nobody is making a hasty decision. It starts, by the way, on the patient's first spoken request to the attending physician for the End of Life Option Act. And then we have a fifteen-day waiting period in which we can't help a patient at all. It assumes patients haven't had forethought before those fifteen days; as if they haven't done a huge amount of contemplating as their illness has progressed. I haven't met a patient who hasn't thought about this for a long time before he or she comes to me with the first request. And many of these patients die during the fifteen-day waiting period, in exactly the way they don't want to. I've seen many patients die during the waiting period, and this is consistent with all the Oregon data over twenty years. About one-third of our patients have died during the fifteen-day waiting period. This is a badly written piece of the legislation. I think this requirement needs to go.

D: Tell me about your experience when an individual has gone through the entire process, and how you as the medical doctor are with that patient at the end.

DR. S: Our practice has a fundamental belief that this is the most difficult experience for patients in their lifetimes and for their families. It's complex. Death is complex and death is important. We don't tell the patient, "Here's the prescription, take it when you're ready." We stay involved as much as possible, because when the patient is ready is not always clear. And we want to be there and have this complex conversation about whether to take the medication. Maybe they're just having a good death anyway, and they don't need it. We help them with that decision as well. But if they decide to take the aid-in-dying medication, the question is when? Do I wait another week? Do I take it now because I may get sicker? Do I wait until my family visits? All of these things are part of the discussion.

And then, the day a patient takes the medication is an anxiety-ridden day, a very, very difficult day for a family. Commonly, they're left alone without any professional help for this. We don't believe in that. As part of our practice, we're there at the bedside on the day. We're there to talk with the family, make sure that everybody's okay, explain to them what the process is. This is a medical procedure, and we don't want people to be left alone with it.

We stay to help administer the medications. We don't give the medications. The law says the patient has to self-administer, so certainly the patient will ingest the medications. But there's preparation involved.

We also watch the patient and describe to him or her what will happen. The whole family needs to know what they'll be seeing. What will Mom or Dad look like as they become unconscious? How long will it take to become unconscious? Will they be suffering after they're asleep? Can they still hear? What is their heart doing now? It seems they've been unconscious for twenty minutes and their heart is still going — why is that?

We know these deaths can take anywhere from ten minutes to ten hours. There are some reports we've had from Oregon of three to four days. So you don't leave a family alone with that. That's not good medicine. A trained person has to be there at the bedside. In the future, I would love for it to be a hospice nurse. We don't think that families should be alone when they do this.

D: That's very comforting to know. Please talk about the problems with Seconal.

DR. S: Got another two hours? Seconal

has been the medicine that's traditionally been used in Oregon. It's a barbiturate; it puts people to sleep, deeply enough that they usually stop breathing, so that you're suppressing the brain, which drives respiration to a significant enough extent that breathing stops. Seconal is a very, very good drug. But it's not necessarily reliable. When you read the Oregon data, you see that there have been ten-minute deaths and that the median death lasts about two hours. That all looks great until you look at the extremes and you hear about the four-day deaths. Which means that Seconal does not reliably suppress respiration. One of the advantages of having a new state and a bigger state than Oregon take another look at this is to review the use of Seconal. We did not want to accept a medication that is not consistent enough for our needs, let alone the fact that its price has gone up to $3,500 a dose. And it's not covered by insurance. So, we have a price issue and a quality issue.

D: And forgive me for bringing up such a mundane factor, but isn't there also a taste issue?

DR. S: Every one of the aid-in-dying medications, because we use such high dosages, has a taste issue. They're all equally unpalatable.

D: What about the European model? Can you comment on that? I read a while back about the 104-year-old man who lived in Australia and had to fly to Switzerland because he wanted aid in dying. Tell me what you know about what happens in Switzerland and whether you think that approach to medical aid in dying is something you as a physician might aspire to.

DR. S: We don't have to go as far as Switzerland; we can just travel across the border to Canada to see a better model than ours. In California, and in every state that's passed a law, we are restricted to medicines taken by mouth. And the intention of that, trying to be gracious to the legislators, has been that it is a final consent. You put that medicine in your hand, you swallow it, that is guaranteeing to the degree you can that the patient has consented to the medication. That, to me, is about as rational as saying, "We have your permission to take out your appendix, thank you for your permission, here's a scalpel, please do it." We don't need that final consent in medicine.

Let me focus on the issue of swallowing medications. The legislature, in an attempt at wisdom, was saying they want to know that there's a final consent from the patient at that moment; that no one is being coerced or forced to do this, or we haven't slipped into so-called euthanasia. So we ask patients to drink the medicine, showing their final consent.

I can't begin to tell you how many problems that brings on. Number one: when patients are really, really ill, so are their guts, their intestines. They don't absorb medications very well. When you see frail old patients dying of cancer, and they've wasted away, so have their intestines, and so the oral route doesn't work for them. Second, we have issues with how much medicine they can take. Then we have issues with some patients, such as ALS patients, who don't have the strength to take the medication. And I as a doctor have to tell you how silly and uncomfortable I feel sitting at a patient's bedside, knowing I have a complex medical procedure to stop some-one's heart, and that all I'm allowed to do is provide liquid medications to swallow, when I have a nice IV nearby and he or she can sign a consent form at that moment and let me do it the right way.

The right way would be the most successful way. For some patients, it might be the oral route. For some patients, it could be via feeding tube. For some it would be intravenously. For some patients, it might even be by rectal administration. But the point is, I can look at a patient and say, "You are this weak and about to lose your ability to swallow. You're not going to be able to do it in two days." Therefore, because of the legislation, patients are going to die a week before they wanted to, because otherwise they're going to lose their ability to swallow.

I think if the legislature is insistent on the oral route as the final permis-sion, let's go along and fulfill every part of the law with the oral route, and the patient swallows the medications. But if the patient's heart has not stopped four hours later, and the fam-ily is waiting and wondering what's happening, I would like to have the right to do what I can do as a doctor, which is to start an intravenous line and give IV medications to end the patient's life. I consider any death longer than five hours to be a failure of aid in dying because that's torture for the family to wait that long. What I would like is for the legislature to understand that, by mandating the oral route, they've created either failed aid in dying or very long aid in dying.

D: I have finally a very difficult issue to take up with you. I, at eighty-one years old, have decided and told my family that should I move toward Alzheimer's and if I am no longer of use to society, when I can no longer care for myself, when I can no longer relate to those around me, I wish to end my life. Do you believe that is a legitimate request to make, and one that would eventually be accepted in the law?

DR. S: My personal belief is that with the right stringent regulations of what has to happen and very specific outlines of what criteria you have to meet at the time, then yes, I believe aid in dying should be allowed to happen under that circumstance. That said, my personal belief means nothing. I don't think society is in agreement yet. I don't think states are ready to sanction that. I think we're at the beginning of understanding aid in dying for people with a terminal illness who can speak for themselves. And I think that we will move slowly, because of necessity we have to on these issues.

We get calls regularly from families of people with dementia who want to know what we can do. And somebody who is at the edge of sometimes being coherent and sometimes not, do we catch that person at the coherent times, and let that person say he or she would like aid in dying, and let that count? And if they're coherent on the day of their death and can self-administer, have we complied with the law? Well, technically, yes, but I'm not comfortable doing it yet. Some people might say we're moving down a slippery slope, toward abuse, and others might say we're moving toward the fact that this is an appropriate way for people to want to die. This is a question of a patient's autonomy in decision making, and I think that's a good thing.

DEBORAH GATZEK KRATTER

ATTORNEY AT LAW, A PATIENT OF
DR. LONNY SHAVELSON'S

DIANE: Debbie, tell me about yourself and your illness.

DEBORAH KRATTER: I was diagnosed with pancreatic cancer in early 2017. I initially suspected it was something totally unrelated, waited a little too long to get my diagnosis. But when I did, I got a call from the doctor saying they had reviewed the CT scan and I have pancreatic cancer, and it looks like it's spread. I immediately went on the Internet to find out what was going on, and was dismayed to see how bad the prognosis was. It's usually four to six months.

D: Tell me what you were doing at the time you got the diagnosis. Were you still practicing as an attorney?

DK: I was. I was still a member of the bar association, although retired from my primary occupation. I was very active on the board of a public company, on the audit committee, head of nominating and corporate governance. I was on the board of directors of the home-owners' association where I'm living now. And I was involved with some other charitable organizations. I was a pretty active person.

D: When you received the diagnosis and began researching on your own and saw the prognosis, what were your first reactions?

DK: My reaction was that I did not want to go through what it looked like I was going to go through. I have to preface that by saying that I had pretty much been an advocate for end-of-life options for a long time, having seen a couple of family members go through unpleasant situations. My thought was: What do I do to make this easier on myself?

D: Did you talk with your own physicians about not wanting to have the end of your life be difficult?

DK: Ultimately, I did. But the first thing I did was research, because I had remembered hearing that California had recently adopted the end-of-life option, so my first research was on how to get it. Then I spoke with my primary-care physician, who was pretty sympathetic. By that time I was involved in a university health-care system that specialized in oncology, and ran into more roadblocks.

D: What kinds of roadblocks?

DK: Initially, they did not seem to know how to make it happen, even though I went online, downloaded all the forms, and said, "Okay, here they are, I qualify, let's do this." And they really didn't know how to handle it. They were surprised I was asking for it at that point and argued with me about asking for it. It took me a couple of months of kind of — I don't want to say "nasty" — but unpleasant interactions. I was under a lot of stress in trying to make this happen.

D: What were they saying to you?

DK: They were like, "Why do you want to do this now? Why do you want to start this process? We don't know how your treatment is going to work. There are all sorts of palliative treatments we can consider. You could go on hospice, you can be put on higher and higher doses of morphine." I kept saying, "I want to be in control, and I want the comfort of knowing I'm in control." I think they initially thought I was a suicidal person. So I made it clear that I'm not suicidal. I just want to continue to be me, to be the active person I am. And if I am a person in bed all day, that's not me. But there was a certain amount of discomfort on their part.

D: I gather you then set out to find a doctor who would help you. How did you find Dr. Lonny Shavelson?

DK: I went on the Internet to check whether there were any doctors who specialized in the California end-of-life option, and thank God I found Lonny, the perfect person to help me through this. When we first met, we didn't know that we would be here a year later. But it just made me feel so much more comfortable, going through the chemo and all of the stuff, knowing that if, at some point, I really can't take this anymore, I have control. I have options.

D: Can you tell me how many chemotherapy treatments you've had? This yearlong process has taken you into areas you had no idea you'd be in.

DK: Yeah, I had heard of chemotherapy, never knew what it was. The first treatment I received was relatively gentle. It worked well for I think six cycles, which was once a week for three weeks and then off one week. It worked very well, but after six cycles, it stopped working. Then they put me on a second, much tougher regime, and I'm still on it. A cancer researcher I know calls it the "sledgehammer." That requires me to be at an infusion center for six hours at a time, and then they hook me up to a portable pump, but that's a joke because it's a two-pound battery-operated pump that I have to wear for forty-eight hours. If you can imagine being tethered to something for forty-eight hours, so when you sleep, you have to subconsciously be aware of how you're moving. I've gone through twelve cycles of that and it's working well, and I have more cycles scheduled.

D: What have been your physical reactions to this chemotherapy?

DK: What I first noticed is a tingling in my hands. It makes me less adept at doing things like putting on a necklace. Earrings are almost impossible. Fortunately, I can still use my computer. The other weird thing is a neuropathy in my feet; it feels like I'm walking on sand. I keep thinking, Did I go on the beach and I didn't know it?

D: So you have to be very careful as you walk?

DK: You bring up another point. All these chemo drugs are really bad on lots of parts of your body, including your bones. And since I've started on the chemo, I've had three bone fractures in my feet.

The first time I asked whether this was related to the chemo, I got a shrug. And the second time, when it was in my right foot, which prevented me from driving, I asked again and got another shrug. So, I went back on the Internet and discovered there were studies that clearly showed this to be a well-known side effect and that it's best to treat people for it. And I had not been treated. Even now, no one is offering to do something. I have to say, I can imagine that if I had a fracture in both feet at the same time, I would be calling Lonny. I can't imagine that I would be in that situation when you know you can't heal and then the next time you put your foot down and you want to take a little walk, you can't.

One of the important things about me is that I'm a very avid exerciser. Since I can't exercise, I can't hike, and I can't take long walks, it really drives me crazy.

D: So let's bring in Dr. Lonny Shavelson, who is the person you found with joy because he gave you that control over your life.

DK: My hero.

D: Lonny, how unusual a patient is Debbie, having had a diagnosis of pancreatic cancer and having learned that the time she had left would likely be short?

DR. SHAVELSON: I have to say that a prognosis is always taken with a grain of salt. It's like looking at any actuarial table; you think you have the data to support it, and then, there are people who are going to exceed our expectations. I think in this case, the prognosis, in essence, was inaccurate. The first thought is that a person with pancreatic cancer that has spread will not survive more than four to six months. What some of the critics of the law say is that we aren't good at making prognoses, and the fact is, it is a vague science. But that doesn't necessarily harm us with the End of Life Option Act. (to Deborah) You knew you had the option. Were you harmed by living longer?

DK: Not at all. I think having this option made me more open to trying treatment, even though I knew it might be very unpleasant. I'll try this, I'll try that, and see how it goes. And if I can't take it, I have a place to go. It actually made me more open to alternatives, and able to live longer, by having the option available to me.

D: Deborah, can you take us back to the first time you met Lonny?

DK: Lonny came to the house and was so much the opposite of what I had experienced, open to and supportive of what I was going through, and he explained fully how the process would work. It was like the shutters being opened. It was wonderful.

D: What did he explain to you about how the process would work?

DK: How it would be at the end. Also, Lonny told me that not only would he be the prescriber, but he would be there at the time that I was actually ready to make the final decision. It's not like I have the pills in my cupboard and if I have a bad day, I might just run upstairs and take them. I know I have to call Lonny and he will be there and probably ask me some questions about how long I've been feeling this way, and that if I say it's been going on for a long time, Lonny will get here as fast as he's able. Or he might say, "Let's give it another couple of days, why don't we, and see how you feel." I feel really comfortable that he would be doing what he thinks is best. It's not mechanical at all. There's a lot of empathy.

D: Have you called him?

DK: No, in fact I've been at the far right end of the bell curve as far as doing well. And what's been very, very nice is that Lonny and his office keep checking in with me to see how I'm doing.

DR. S: One of our principles is that we continue to follow patients. We really want to know our patients, because we're going to participate, at some point, in a very important day in their lives. But I have to ask you again, Deborah, because I'm still curious, was there any harm done in your receiving a less-than-six-months prognosis? You lived longer, and it's wonderful to be here with you. Did we lose anything by starting the process sooner?

DK: No, not a bit. I gained a much higher quality of life throughout the treatment. I gained the knowledge that I wasn't afraid to undergo the treatment. It's been 100 percent positive knowing that I have the option and that I can take chances, and if something doesn't work, I'm not stuck with that choice. In fact, I would love to get some of the doctors to think outside the box a little more.

DR. S: You know, the opposition to this law would say that by giving you this option so soon, there was a risk you might have taken it prematurely. Is there any truth that there was a risk of your making a mistake, taking the medication and dying, when you actually could have lived for a year?

DK: You made it so clear that this was something that would be a very thoughtful process. I wanted this from the very beginning because I wanted to be in control. I wanted the comfort that comes with knowing I'm in control. So, no negatives whatsoever.

D: When I walked into your lovely home

today, one of the first things I set eyes on was the grandchild's table you had set up right here in your family room and just outside your kitchen area. That made me wonder how your family and friends feel about your making that decision to be in control, to say at some point, to Lonny and to yourself and to your family and friends: Now is the time.

DK: My family is uniformly supportive. Each one has slightly different concerns. My son, whose child gets the benefit of the room here, is concerned that my grandchild may have noticed something. There've been some questions about whether they will be here when it happens, and I'm not sure. Actually, I don't think I want an audience. My daughter is very pragmatic and understands 100 percent. My husband's attitude is more that he knows this is what I want to do, but doesn't want to talk about it. And my friends, many of whom at my age still have elderly parents, have been completely supportive and said, "I would want to do the same thing." And friends whose spouses have died have expressed the wish they could have had the option for their spouses.

D: How does the fact that your husband says he understands but doesn't want to talk about it make you feel?

DK: It's who my husband has been his whole life. He's not an emotion sharer. It's not a surprise, and it doesn't really reflect on this situation.

D: I'm concerned about the bones in your feet. If you couldn't navigate on your own and would have to be, say, wheelchair-bound or even bedridden, would that be a deciding factor?

DK: At this point, I think it might be. If both feet were broken at the same time, it would make me feel like what's the point of continuing on with the chemotherapy, which is not a pleasant thing to go through. It would just make me think that to keep on doing this only so that I can stay in bed . . . that wouldn't be who I am.

D: And at that point would you turn to Lonny?

DK: I may well.

D: And, Lonny, how would you react?

DR. S: We would have quite a long conversation.

D: Tell me about that conversation.

DR. S: I'm going to preface this by saying that if you and I would disagree about this, in the end the choice is still yours. But I might argue with you. I would say, "Let's see if we can work around this disability." Will using a wheelchair be as bad as you think it will be? Maybe not. What can we do that could help you while you still have some quality of life left, and let's talk about what *quality of life* means. If it means being able to work, well, there are computers that can work in wheelchairs. If it means getting ramps for your house, well, then maybe we can get you outside, since you like being active. I would make some pretty strong arguments for finding some adaptive measures. But I'd then say that, if you think about this and you're persistent and, in the end, this is what you want, and I'm convinced it's not just your depression talking, I'm going to respect your wishes.

D: Everything you talked about that could be done — all of that costs a great deal of money. What happens when an individual comes to you without resources?

DR. S: The easiest example, the most common red line that people tell me they'll never cross, and when they'll be ready to die, is being in bed wearing diapers. I hear that a lot. And then the time comes, and they're in bed, and they now need diapers. But after pooping in the bed without diapers for a couple of days, they're so grateful to have those diapers. Then they live on for weeks with the diapers. They adjust. This is what we call the moving line in the sand. Diapers are not very expensive. Ramps and robotic exoskeletons are. Generally, we find ways to make people more comfortable as they die which are not expensive in the first place.

But your point is well taken, which is that people with fewer resources don't get as good medical care. That is sadly true at the end of life, as it is during life. I don't know if we can solve that problem. We do the best that we possibly can. But wheelchairs are not that hard to get, ramps are really not that hard to get. I think hospice works very well if there is increased disability when someone is dying. The question is: What is that real line in the sand that patients won't cross? That's the time when they're ready for aid in dying. And typically, we've crossed a number of lines in the sand along the way, and they have adjusted.

D: Tell me how much it costs when an individual comes to you and asks for help.

DR. S: Our practice strongly believes that nobody should be denied this because of lack of funds, so we have a sliding scale that starts at the top and goes all the way to zero, which we apply not infrequently. There's a flat fee of $2,600 for anybody who wants to avail themselves of our services, from the initial visit and on through the entire process, which sometimes lasts a year, and ends with my being there at the bedside. With some people, it's one week. We see them one week and we help them die the next week. So it's quite variable as to how long it takes, but there's one fee for everyone, $2,600, and if people don't have the funds, we'll slide that down as low as is necessary.

D: Dr. Shavelson, tell me how typical a patient Debbie is.

DR. S: Totally atypical. Most of the patients we see when they're very close to death, they've been in hospice, or we bring them into hospice right away because they are so close to death. I would guess we see most of our patients within four to ten weeks of the time they die, whether by aid in dying or by other processes. They're quite ill. We're the practice of last resort. They've usually tried their own doctors and been turned away. And they've tried their university care center or their oncologist and been turned away. When they find us, the first thing we ask is what care they've been getting, because we want to keep patients on the same regimen. When we take patients on, it's often because they have not been able to find another doctor who's been willing to work with them.

D: Deborah, what happened when your own doctor found out you had turned to Lonny?

DK: My primary-care physician was very supportive and happy that I'd found Lonny. The doctors at the university care system seemed a bit miffed that I was asking for this procedure at the point I was asking for it, and I still have a feeling that with one particular physician — it's hard to say it's a resentment, but there's just surprise.

"You see, you were wrong, because you're still here." That's because he did not understand that my whole point was not that I wanted to die then; I just wanted the comfort of knowing that when I cross my red line, I get to cross it and I don't have to wait for somebody else to say, "No, there's a further red line that we want you to cross."

D: Deborah, do you know what your red line is?

DK: I think I do, but I suspect I don't. When I think of the whole idea of chemotherapy and all I've gone through, and how I thought, No, I'm not going to do that, and all the times when I'm hooked up to this portable pump, the day after the steroids wear off (which give you a bit of a high), and all I'm left with is being hooked up to this pump I'm carrying around, there are times I think, This is just really crazy. But two or three days later, I'm back, handling a board meeting.

D: Debbie, when the time comes and you reach what you feel is the red line, how sure are you that you'll use the medication when Lonny provides it?

DK: I am pretty certain I will. In part because, for the past few decades, I've had a very bad back and a lot of pain, and I know how much pain I can take and continue on. And if the time comes when there's pain and discomfort and nobody's benefiting from it, I'm not doing anything to raise a small child, I'm not doing anything for anybody else, I can't think right now of any way where I'd say, "Yeah, I'll take another few days of pain." That's not quality of life. I am pretty certain that before I get there, I will be in touch with Lonny.

D: And when you do receive that medication, do you know what it will be, and how you will take it?

DK: Lonny made that very clear. While I don't know the chemical names, the first two drugs put you to sleep pretty quickly, and then there are the drugs that I have to take myself that will ultimately slow the action of the heart. Lonny even made clear this is not something that will necessarily happen in a matter of minutes, that some patients are a bit more resistant and may be alive longer than one might hope. But I feel 100 percent fully informed.

D: So if you do receive that medication, I gather you'd prefer to be alone? At least right now, that's your thinking? In my own case, I think what I'd like to do is to have my family, my closest friends, and perhaps then go off to my bedroom. I would hope a physician would be there to guide me, perhaps my own daughter, who is a physician, plus my son, and my husband. But you think you'd rather be alone?

DK: Well, I think the first part, the predeparture party — It's funny you mention that. There's a wonderful episode on *Grace and Frankie.*

D: Wasn't it wonderful?

DK: Absolutely wonderful episode, where she gave herself a wonderful going-away party. But I think that's an unusual situation, where somebody would be that well and be able to have a fun party and then go upstairs. I have a feeling that I will not be that well at the point when I make the decision. As for whether I would want my family or friends around, I haven't given it a lot of thought. A lot of my thinking is about how it would affect other people. I don't think I would want to put my family in the position of being upstairs in the bedroom waiting to see when I stop breathing. I think that might be unpleasant for them. At the very end, I don't think I want an audience.

D: Lonny, have all the people who've come to you been Caucasian?

DR. S: No. The smallest percentage have been African Americans, and I think probably rightly so, out of their distrust of the medical system. We've had a surprisingly significant higher percentage than I would have expected of Asians in our practice. And we've had a high, significant number of Latinos. But I think that access to good medical care — and I consider aid in dying to be access to good medical care — is still more available to privileged, educated white people. So we see the same skewing in our practice that you see in oncology practices, early mammograms, and vaccinations. We see that imbalance across the scale of medicine.

The common accusation is that this is just for rich white people. It's for people who can get on a computer, find a doctor who will be cooperative and help them get what they want —

and those tend to be the more affluent people who expect more privileges in all aspects of medicine, including ours. And yet, I've been surprised. Because we are in California, we don't have a predominantly white population. We have quite a variety. I have to say that the shortage has been in African Americans. I don't think the medical establishment has been good at building trust with the African American community.

D: Some opponents of medical aid in dying fear that there's a slippery slope, that there could come a time when the disabled, perhaps the mentally challenged, might be taken against their will. How do you respond to that kind of concern, Lonny?

DR. S: I think we have to be a somewhat evidence-based society. And in twenty-two years of practice in Oregon, and now in California, in Washington, and in many other states, there haven't been any documented cases of that type of abuse. Given their intensity, the opponents of the law would have pointed out "slippery-slope" transgressions by now, if there were any. We've stuck to the law, we've followed the law, we've worked with the types of patients for whom the laws were intended. And I think that if there's argument about whether we will ever have this with patients with dementia, or with patients who are severely disabled, I think that those are valid questions. Society has to answer those questions. As of now, what we have is a law that says we work with terminally ill patients. We follow that law. I am very, very careful when I see, for example, a Parkinson's patient who is severely disabled, but not yet terminal. I have to turn those patients down, although they make very intense requests, being ready to end their lives. This law does not apply to patients who are severely disabled; it applies to patients who are terminal. There are hard discussions, but we follow the law.

DR. DAVID GRUBE

NATIONAL MEDICAL DIRECTOR,
COMPASSION & CHOICES

*A Lecture to Second-Year Medical Students
George Washington University,
April 15, 2019*

Our topic today is medical aid in dying. I give lectures about this topic all across the nation, but my favorite audience is medical students, and my favorite, favorite audience is first- and second-year medical students.

I practiced for thirty-five years in a little town in Oregon. In Oregon, we've had this law for almost twenty-two years, and here in D.C., you've had it for a little over a year. By the time you graduate from medical school, many states will have this option for choice at the end of life. And that's why I think it's important for you to learn about it.

The first thing to remember is that the annual mortality rate does not change. I think it's important to remind ourselves that death is not the enemy — we're all going to die. The enemy is terminal suffering, suffering at the very, very end of life.

There are now nine jurisdictions in the United States that allow medical aid in dying, and if you add up all the people who live in those places, that's about one in five Americans who have aid in dying as an option at the end of their lives. Oregon was the first, and New Jersey just came on board.

Aid in dying essentially applies to an individual, your patient, who has to be an adult, has to be a resident of the state where you practice, has to have the capacity to understand what they're doing. It's not for people with dementia or people having difficulty understanding informed consent. They have to have volition. That means, it's their choice. No one can choose for them. And they have to have a terminal diagnosis. That means, they have to have six months or fewer to live, such as a hospice patient, if you will.

And *self-ingestion* means that the patient takes the medicine himself or herself.

There are protections. Because it is a law, it is something that you, as a doctor (in a few years), cannot be sued for. Indeed, no doctor has ever been sued in the states where medical aid in dying is authorized.

And there has never been any disciplinary action against a doctor. I sat on the Oregon Medical Board for many years, and each year we would look at cases, but we never took any disciplinary action if the doctor acted in good faith in accordance with the provisions of the law.

There are also important protections for the patient. If people choose this option, it doesn't have any impact on their life insurance policies or any other contracts they may have. If people choose this, their death certificate does not state the cause of death to be medical aid in dying; it states the disease that was responsible for the end of life, such as lung cancer, ALS, et cetera. There are two parts to a death certificate: the legal part, which is for your estate planning and so on, and the medical part, which is for epidemiology.

All the data about aid in dying are collected on forms a doctor fills out. This is an intimate and private experience. And most important, it does not constitute suicide, or euthanasia, or mercy killing, or homicide. I can say that to you clinically, but it's in every state law as well. It can't be called those things because it isn't those things.

We've had this law for a long time in Oregon, and I think we've had some unexpected results. First of all, we didn't realize that just having the conversation about aid in dying is palliative in and of itself. Many patients who are dying wanted to talk. And after we talked, they could have — but usually did not — choose it. They felt better knowing that I would listen to them. I would be available for them. I would not abandon them. I would not brush this off as a silly thought they were having. I would not question why they wanted to talk about it.

Another interesting thing is that most people do not choose aid in dying because of extreme pain. Everybody thinks, Well, gosh, they're suffering because they're in all this pain. No, their suffering is not necessarily pain. Their suffering may be anhedonia — lack of joy or lack of pleasure, loss of autonomy, loss of dignity, when you have to have someone else clean you up every day, you can't take care of yourself, or you're incontinent. Pain comes in about fifth or sixth on a list of reasons people give for wanting aid in dying.

And, very importantly, this is not something that people have taken advantage of. Minority groups, the disabled, the poor, are not people who are ever coerced into this. That just doesn't happen. Some of the people opposed to medical aid in dying say, "Well, this is going to be against the disabled." Absolutely not, and that's not the case in any state, including Oregon. It's about people who are about to die. They may or may not have a disability, but it's not about their disability, it's about their coming death.

It's important for you to know that of the people who go through the process, only two-thirds of them end of up taking the medication. Fully a third who have a prescription don't take it. They just want the option. They want to be empowered to have a choice. They have no choice about being about to die, but they would like to have certain other choices.

It's also important to realize that assisted dying is not a very common occurrence in Oregon. We have about 35,000 deaths every year, and last year 170 people took the medication — about 0.2 percent of our deaths. This ratio holds true in other states as well.

This is a really important part of the conversation. I think you may have noticed, I have not called medical aid in dying "suicide" — it's also called "voluntary assisted dying" or "physician-assisted dying" — we don't use the word *suicide* because it's *not* suicide. It's a completely different situation. I, unfortunately, early in my practice, was called to the home of a patient of mine, a hospice patient. I walked into the bedroom, and he had taken a shotgun and put it into his mouth and pulled the trigger. I still have nightmares about that experience. It was terrible for me, and for my wife, who came over to help, to clean, to take care of his widow and their family. It was a horrible thing.

In contrast, I attended a planned death eight days ago, where a woman who was dying of a peritoneal carcinomatosis had her seven grandchildren there at her bedside, her kids, her dog, her own music. It was a beautiful, serene death, peaceful, the family all together. They were sad that she died, but they were happy she was no longer suffering. These are two completely different situations.

Suicide is an epidemic in our society, one we need to spend more resources on preventing. A suicide is often an impulse act and the person who commits it has some kind of mental illness. These people have PTSD, they have addictive personality trait, they have major depressive disorder or whatever. Aid-in-dying patients are the opposite of impulsive. They have planned this, they have thought it out. They have the support of their families. They're with their families. And so the grief reaction after aid in dying is normal, whereas a grief reaction to a suicide is terrible for the family, for the loved ones, and for the medical team, too.

B. J. Miller is a fellow I know, a hospice doctor. He talks about how the language we use at end of life is so important — that we don't ever use language that causes shame or fear or guilt or anxiety for the person who is dying. We want to use kind, and not hurtful, language. And that's why calling what we are doing "aid in dying" is really different from calling it "suicide."

As I've said, only a quarter of the people who consider aid in dying as an end-of-life option use it because they don't have adequate pain control. That's been a huge, wonderful change in the forty years I've practiced medicine. But we can't always manage intolerable suffering. And who defines suffering? It's the patient who defines suffering, it's not the doctor. That's really important to remember.

Historically, most people who use aid in dying have been cancer patients. But more often now we're seeing other kinds of things creep in. For instance, ALS, which is a terrible disease. It's always fatal and it always results in complete body paralysis. Aid in dying is being considered by those patients more frequently. And now terminal emphysema and heart failure patients are doing so as well. One of the patients for whom I prescribed medication had terminal emphysema. She'd been on and off a ventilator, she had had pneumonia over and over again. She was on oxygen, she couldn't even get out of bed. She was being smothered. Every moment, she was being smothered. It was terrible. She had a terrible experience at the end of life, and she chose aid in dying.

To go back: When I came to medical school in Oregon, the enemy for me was death. I was going to cure everybody I saw. I was going to learn as much as I could, so that I could be the best doctor and go do that. And one of the things I did learn in medical school was that death is not the enemy. All of us are going to die, and there are many wonderful things that you, as future doctors, can do that will assuage people's diseases and make them healthier.

The enemy, again, is terminal suffering, when you have just a few days left to live and you're having pain that's intolerable. When I have conversations with people who are opposed to aid in dying, and I ask them how anybody could be in favor of suffering at the end of life, how could anyone support that, they generally agree with me.

There are two things that matter in end-of-life care: comforting our patients, and respecting their wishes. We take care of people, we never abandon them. We honor their choices. It's not about us, it's about them. That's what aid in dying is about — honoring people's choices, preventing suffering, and comforting individuals at the end of life.

QUESTIONS FROM STUDENTS

About fifty second-year medical students attended Dr. Grube's lecture. They sat in a large auditorium, chatting loudly with one another before the lecture began. There were more women than men, from many races and ethnicities, all dressed casually.

STUDENT: So, when discussing different options with patients, how do you go about approaching this as an option? Is it as soon as a terminal diagnosis is made, as soon as you sense that a patient is open to this sort of option? Do you bring it up or does the patient?

DR. G: What a great question! It depends, of course. Most of these people have been sick for a long time, and about 95 percent of these people are in hospice. They've been through years of chemotherapy and many surgeries. Most of them aren't naïve about the situation.

A good palliative-care physician asks questions like "How do you conceive of or perceive your last day? Where do you want to be? Do you want to be in the hospital?" Some people want to be. "If we can get you there, do you want to be at home with your loved ones? Do you want to plan your death? Do you want to have it at a time you choose? Do you want hospice?" All those kinds of questions.

The reality is, the patients bring it up. Almost never do you have to say, "Well, now you can do palliative care, you can do terminal sedation, you can do deep sedation, you can do voluntary stopping of eating and drinking." It isn't like that. It's more like getting to where they are. What are their fears? What are their anxieties? How can we deal with those feelings?

STUDENT: If the patient makes the decision that this is something they want to do, and they get the medica-

tions, how often do they use the medication versus deciding not to?

DR. G: About half the people who begin
the process die before they get through
it. These are protections that we have;
there's a waiting period of two weeks,
and you have to see two different doctors, and sign paperwork. There are
different protections, so that people
don't just do this willy-nilly. Average
length of time to go through the process is a month, and about half the
people die before that.

STUDENT: How do states that don't
allow medical aid in dying justify the
idea that palliative care is so much better than medical aid in dying? From
what I know of palliative care, if someone is truly suffering, doctors will put
them in almost a comatose state until
they pass away naturally. What is the
justification that the states have for
preventing medical aid in dying from
being an option?

DR. G: Continuous deep sedation,
which we used to call "palliative sedation," or "terminal sedation," is a very
high-tech thing. Generally, you've got
to be in a facility; you don't usually do
it at home. It's controlled by the doc-

tor. The doctor puts you to sleep and keeps you asleep until you pass away. It's all really about the doctor rather than the patient.

Continuous deep sedation is legal in all states. The question really is, How could *it* be allowed and not medical aid in dying? And I have no answer. The major opponents to this are religious groups who believe that God put you on the earth and that God's going to take you away. There are also disability groups that have somehow bought into the idea that they might be at risk, when, in fact, that's never been shown to be the case in any state.

STUDENT: I'm kind of confused about the reasons why people choose medical aid in dying. Financial issues are only three percent of the reasons cited. I'm concerned about how there would be a valid reason for someone to go through this process.

DR. G: Maybe that has happened, but it's never been something I've run into. Ninety-eight percent of people who choose aid in dying in the authorized states do have insurance. And our Medicaid, our state insurance, pays for it.

STUDENT: Could you tell us about the medications that are actually used for this?

DR. G: The rapid-acting barbiturates have been chosen — pentobarbital and secobarbital. Then pentobarbital was taken away from the U.S. because of some botched capital-punishment case. It's produced in Denmark, and so we don't have it. And then secobarbital was no longer available in the U.S. after January 1, 2019, and no one knows why. So doctors and pharmacists in authorized states have gotten together and come up with two protocols. One is a combination of diazepam (which is Valium), 1 gram; and digitalis, 50 milligrams, which is two thousand times the regular dose; 15 grams of morphine sulfate; and 2 grams of propranolol. That is very effective. It's not as effective as secobarbital or the barbiturates, but it is effective. However, there have been some prolonged deaths with that protocol and particularly with ALS patients, who have really strong hearts when they're thirty-six years old but can't move their bodies and haven't deteriorated physically like a ninety-year-old with lung cancer.

The more up-to-date protocol is called DDMA. It's 100 milligrams of digitalis, and then one half hour later, 1 gram of diazepam, 15 grams of morphine sulfate, and then instead of the propranolol, 8 grams of amitriptyline. That means the death occurs sooner. Rather than lasting an hour or two, it's closer to twenty minutes. That's probably the most commonly used protocol. The complications or the difficulties are that it has to be compounded, and in some places, such as rural Oregon, there aren't compounding pharmacies, so you have to get it from Portland, and that's another barrier and takes more time.

STUDENT: So after a prescription is written and the patient has the medication in hand, what's the process like? Do they set a date, or is it like a ceremony with Grandma and all the grandchildren and the dog?

DR. G: First of all, after the prescription is written I think it's important to tell patients not to fill it until they're absolutely certain they're going to want it. Leave the prescription at the pharmacy.

It doesn't cost them any money and it's safe there. But what happens is all over the board. I'll tell you a very interesting story about a woman who got the prescription. She was dying of cancer, and all of a sudden an experimental treatment came out, and she went to Seattle and got the experimental treatment and lived for four years. She had four really great years. And then the cancer came back and it was horrible. And then she took the medication.

We try to counsel our patients never to take the medication alone, never to take it in a public place, and to tell your family about it. Sometimes family members don't agree and won't participate or get in the way or act out or whatever. But if this person is in hospice, then he or she has the support of the chaplain and the social worker and the nurse's aide, and it's much, much better.

STUDENT: So if it's self-prescribed and self-administered, how can you be sure the pill doesn't fall into the wrong hands?

DR. G: End-of-life patients have a gob of things at their bedside. They have a hospice rescue pack, they have their chemotherapy, their aspirin. All medicine is a poison. When you use the correct amount, it can be therapeutic, but it should be stored securely.

STUDENT: We're fortunate to have physicians like you providing this care for patients, but how can we empower other physicians to seek further training in this area, and also to have these important conversations with palliative-care patients?

DR. G: Through education at an early age, in medical school. I teach in the medical school in Portland, and I always teach the first-year students like you if I can, because you have the most open minds about choices and options. Teaching about the difference between personal beliefs and professional integrity — that's very important. We all have very deep and personal beliefs. But professional integrity means that while you take those into the exam room, there it's about the patients. It's not about you, and you need to respond to their concerns.

I teach in hospices and medical programs, trying to get state medical associations to change, and now I think fourteen or fifteen different state medical associations, as well as the American Academy of Family Medicine, recently reversed their opposition. Now we're working on the American Medical Association. The American Nurses Association is probably going to change their position on this. That's huge because, being married to a nurse with more than forty years of experience, I know where the power lies in medicine. And thank heavens.

STUDENT: Have you worked with other members of the medical team who don't agree with this decision?

DR. G: You never have to. In all states, in all systems, if this is something that you do not personally believe is correct, you can opt out. I'm on the board of directors of a hospice, and we have a policy that supports choice, but if a nurse does not want to participate, we make sure she or he is able to not participate and we have another nurse there instead. That's true about pretty much all policies, and it's very important.

In regard to getting people to understand, I think one way is to state our advance directives, our living wills, and video-record them on our iPads or iPhones. It makes a big difference when you can show that to a loved one and say, "This is what Mom really wanted. See, when she wasn't so sick, she said this." I think that's way better than just having it written down on a piece of paper.

STUDENT: Since the patient has to be able to self-administer the medicine, do you often see patients grappling with the question of when is the right time to take it, because they don't want to be so far down the road that they can't take it on their own?

DR. G: Yes, and particularly ALS patients and particularly with the swallowing. However, self-ingestion does not necessarily mean swallowing. It can mean even getting someone to mix up the medicine so that you can push it into your feeding tube. There's also a thing called a Macy catheter — a rectal catheter — and with it medicine can be administered rectally.

It's really important to talk about the difference between administration and assisting. Assisting can mean mixing up the medicine, going to the store and getting the medicine, holding a cup while someone sucks out of a straw. That's all fine, all legal. But the administering is not legal if you pour the medicine into the person's mouth. But yes, particularly ALS patients get to that point and come up with creative ideas of how they might be able to take the medicine if they can't use their arms.

I've been talking longer than I should have been. I love talking to young people about this because if I just talk to old doctors, most of them would say they still don't think it's right, and maybe only a few would change their minds. I may not have changed anyone's mind here, but I hope I gave you some information. I'm certainly excited about your future in medicine. You're going to have a great career!

GIZAL RACHITI, FRANKIE BURUPHEE, SOMIA MONUPUTI, AND CHARLIE HARTLEY

FOUR STUDENTS WHO ATTENDED DR. GRUBE'S LECTURE

DIANE: First, give me a sense of your takeaway from the lecture you just heard.

GIZAL: Coming into this, I was a little bit unsure of my position on the subject. I was raised Catholic. So it was always, choose life, anything to protect someone's life, and that includes medical aid in dying. I was really moved by the lecture and all the stories Dr. Grube told about people's dignity. My mother has ovarian cancer, and so if she were to choose that option, I would 100 percent support her, because it's her decision; it's every patient's decision.

FRANKIE: I came in thinking, it's always a conflict, between how I was raised, my beliefs, and how I want to treat patients as a doctor. It's always been my belief that patients have the right to make a choice, no matter what. Yet there's always the inner monologue of: Is it the right thing to do? Listening to the lecture really swayed me in the direction of yes, this is the right thing to do, listening to patients is always the right thing to do, and they should have the autonomy to die as they please.

SOMIA: I came in with an open mind, not knowing too much about the details, although it's something that I had thought about before. I come from a Muslim background, and it's a controversial issue there. But the point that it's about suffering, about decreasing terminal suffering, and how well thought out this process is, and how many obstacles there are to make sure people are considering it fully — a lot of that was very persuasive.

CHARLIE: I actually came in fully convinced that this is something a patient should have the right and ability to do. Both my parents dealt with the early loss of their parents. My dad lost his father at a very young age, and my mom lost her mother in her teens. Then her grandmother had ALS and dealt with the consequences of that late in life. I think it's not within our purview as doctors to tell people how they should determine the end of their lives. And this procedure is something that has been shown to be effective and painless and to relieve people of the pressures they're dealing with as they come to their time. It's something they should be fully empowered to do.

SOMIA: I spent a lot of time in college trying to understand death and dying in different cultures. One of the things I took away from the lecture today was that there's a growing movement in the U.S., and I was excited to see that. I've spent time in the Netherlands, and I talked to a lot of people there about the consequences of assistance in dying. I think one of the challenges will be — and Dr. Grube briefly mentioned this — what we do with people who have cognitive decline. I'm hoping we'll be able to make this available to patients who are undergoing that. This is going to be an interesting ethical and medical issue.

FRANKIE: It seems from the way it was laid out that this is a very long process. It takes quite a while for a patient to be able to be approved for this. Some don't get the approval. There are a lot of safeguards in place to make sure that people aren't making the wrong decision.

D: What was the most important thing Dr. Grube said to you about beginning a conversation with a patient, or with someone you love?

GIZAL: My general impression was of an approach of respect and acknowledgment that this person is the one who's experiencing illness and suffering. It's not what I, as a family member or loved one, or physician, think. It's what they think because it's what they are experiencing. So we should be opening the conversation by wanting to listen and hear what the person is saying and not projecting our own judgments or beliefs onto that person.

D: It used to be that a patient would say, "Well, whatever you say, Doctor." Things have changed now, but would you want to accept that responsibility?

SOMIA: I think one of the great things they're teaching us in medical school, and which will hopefully be the norm going forward, is having more collaboration between the patient and physician in care planning. I would see it as my responsibility to inform patients as much as possible about their options. The really difficult question is when people ask you what you would do if you were in my position, and we haven't gotten into a lot of the nitty-gritty of how we as physicians are supposed to respond to that. And that's, again, injecting your personal beliefs into what should be done.

But I think it is part of our responsibility, as part of the medical community, to have those conversations and be bold enough to raise the topic and then say, "This isn't about me, This is about your journey, and you can ask me any questions you want, but this is not something I can decide for you."

Dr. William Toffler

NATIONAL DIRECTOR,
PHYSICIANS FOR COMPASSIONATE CARE;
PROFESSOR EMERITUS,
OREGON HEALTH & SCIENCE UNIVERSITY

Dr. Toffler and I meet in his home in Portland, Oregon. He is tall, slender, and handsome, with short, curly gray hair. Dr. Toffler lost his wife to cancer about five years earlier. We are seated close together in his living room, which is filled with photographs of his wife and children. Before I begin recording our conversation, he mentions details about *my* life, about my late husband, my children, my background, my upbringing, even my dog Maxie, now deceased. He has clearly done a thorough background check of his interviewer.

DR. TOFFLER: It's a privilege and an honor to be with you, Diane.

DIANE: Thank you. Please tell me about Physicians for Compassionate Care.

DR. T: It's an organization dedicated to giving the best of care at the end of life, and affirming the ethic that all human life is inherently valuable.

D: Oregon's right-to-die law has been in effect for twenty-two years now. Tell me your thinking about this law.

DR. T: Well, first, the name of the law, the "right to die" or so-called death with dignity, is not what we're talking about. Diane, you and I and everyone else are terminal. We don't have a *right* to die, we are all *going* to die.

What I'm trying to fight for is the right to life, in a state where we have adopted the model that some lives are less valuable than others. In Oregon, people are offered treatment under some conditions, but under other conditions, they're not. And the state will deny coverage for people like Barbara Wagner, who was a school bus driver who had lung cancer. The cancer recurred. Her oncologist wanted to give her a drug called Tarceva. She wanted the drug, because, statistically, it would increase her chances of being alive in one year by 45 percent.

She gets a letter from her health insurance, CareOregon, denying coverage for this drug, which she wanted and which the doctor wanted to give her. Yet they would pay 100 percent for her assisted suicide under the rubric "pain relief." Talk about misnomers! She was indignant. What right do they have? They'll pay her to die with dignity by suicide, or the lethal dose of medication, but they won't pay for her to extend her life, which she wanted. She was robust. You wouldn't be able to tell that she had cancer. Remarkably, the drug company offered her the drug for free, and would, if she did well for a year, actually continue to provide her with the drug. So it's paradoxical that the drug companies seem to care more about extending her life than the state of Oregon. And this is what I'm worried about, this inherent conflict of interest, where we have money that could be spent on the living, and giving care to people, and that instead gets spent on the solution to suffering by taking an overdose of medication.

I think people who believe in this paradigm are not bad people. My colleague Dr. David Grube is head of the so-called Compassion & Choices. We see the world differently. I believe the solution to suffering is to help the suf-

ferer, to be with the sufferer, to be willing to suffer with the patient. That's
what I've dedicated my life to, over
these last forty years as a doctor.

D: Would you say that, from the outset,
you did not support Oregon's law?

DR. T: Absolutely, I didn't, I don't. I
think it's a huge violation of the integrity of the patient. I use the analogy of
a courtroom, Diane, and I'm your
defense attorney. And then you're a
little puzzled when I walk across the
aisle, and now I'm actually arguing the
case against you, and it's a capital case.
This is where your life is potentially at
risk. And if you don't think *that's* a
conflict of interest, for me to be on
both sides of the fence, if you will, I'm
also the judge who decides which
lawyer is making the better argument.
And if you're *still* not bothered, I'm
also the executioner who carries out
your death sentence.

Many people are not happy with the
death penalty, because we might make
a mistake. There've been lots of cases
when exculpatory DNA evidence
comes to light, and the person is gone.
Doctors don't have crystal-ball-reading
courses in medical school, and we, too,

are sometimes wrong. Every doctor has seen a case in which somebody lived longer than the doctor predicted.

Even so, my late wife, Marlene, asked the doctor, "How much longer?" We both knew her cancer had spread. It started in her uterus, a leiomyosarcoma of the uterus. And then, it was found in her lungs. That was a death sentence, because there is no cure and it's a relatively rare cancer. The doctor gave her his best professional estimate of three to nine months. We were blessed with four times that time. And that time was precious, as you know from your own experience. Every day is special. And because we see the decline, we know it's not going to be forever, and it changes everything. I think we had only one argument in the last five years of her life, which was a very different amount of arguing from what we had in the previous thirty-five years of marriage. I wouldn't trade a nanosecond of those last years with Marlene.

You know, ending your life isn't rocket science. Seventy thousand people take their lives every year. These are non-assisted suicides. The sad thing is that we as a medical profession are acting like vending machines. There are a million doctors in the country, Diane, and sadly they don't all have the same reverence for life in all its stages.

D: Tell me then, what are the greatest flaws in the Oregon law as you see them?

DR. T: We're dichotomizing the worth of people. We're saying some lives are not worth living. We actually think, as doctors, we're helping the person out, doing something that in at least forty-one other states isn't legal yet. And I'm doing my best to educate people that maybe this isn't a good path to go down.

We've had people who've had something to gain, who stood to gain the house and $90,000, and they've helped somebody to do this. And yes, there are people who are well-intentioned, good people, like my colleague Dr. Grube, but I've never asked a patient (and I doubt that David has either), "What's your life insurance policy? Who's the beneficiary? What ulterior motive might someone have?"

One of my colleagues in this effort to

stop the metastases of this paradigm is Margaret Dore, who is an elder-abuse lawyer in Seattle. She knows that one out of ten elders are abused, and this is not good. The ultimate act of elder abuse is to end the person's life for some secondary gain. It might not even be money. It might be only that the patient is feeling like they're a burden, which is one of the chief reasons why people do this. Their loved ones feel they're a burden.

D: As I understand from the research, Oregon has not reported problems with the elderly being coerced or any incidents of abuse — not only elder abuse, but of any individual being forced to take the medication. Indeed, we've been told that some one-third of those who receive the medication do not use it. I'd be interested in whether you believe those reports to be false. Or do you think abuse or coercion is simply not being reported?

DR. T: Doctors are not present when the overdose is taken, 84 percent of the time, so all the reports are second-hand at best. I grant you that most people do not have bad intentions, but there are some who do. We also know that a study done by one of my colleagues at Oregon Health & Science University, Linda Ganzini, showed that, of the people receiving overdoses, 25 percent (because she was able to give formal psychiatric interviews) met the criteria for major depressive disorder, and 23 percent met the criteria for anxiety disorder. None were diagnosed with those problems by the physicians who gave them the overdose. She, being a neutral person, said that this may put people at risk.

There's never been an investigation of any of these assisted suicides in the state of Oregon, none. The head of the Oregon Health Authority that tracks the data was, for years, Dr. Katrina Hedberg, one of my former medical students who was also in practice with me. She said the department has neither the authorization nor the funding to investigate.

I've had three or four dozen people talk to me about this subject in my practice. I don't want to be pejorative toward doctors who disagree with me. But if I simply go with someone's wishes, without having a dialogue — and I'm not saying that other doctors don't always do this . . . but I can tell you, when 25 percent of the people in a study of some fifty or sixty people weren't diagnosed with their underlying mental disorder by my colleagues, I obviously know that a lot of people aren't asking the right questions.

D.: Do any of your patients come to you saying, "I've had enough"? And how do you deal with that?

DR. T: Sure. I've been taking care of a patient. She's had a lot of disabling problems. She's a very able-bodied person, but she's had a lot of calamities in her life.

She's said this to me many times. Just this week, she's feeling pretty despondent. I basically do what I did with other patients over the years. I mobilize. We've had to redouble our efforts to help this person to reflect on her worth. I've been through this with her many times, and never would I encourage her sense of "It's hopeless, I don't have any reason to live anymore," something she's said to me repeatedly.

Because she happens to have me as a doctor, it's changed the course of her treatment. I'm not speaking as a special person. I'm speaking as somebody who believes in the inherent value of all people's lives, regardless of whether they're distressed or despondent or feel they're a burden. I want to make sure they know that they're not a burden.

D: What if a patient comes to you with what we call "intractable pain," and you then refer them to a palliative-care specialist, and the palliative care does not seem to alleviate the pain? What do you do then?

DR. T: To begin with, not having good pain relief is often touted as the reason for assisted suicide. Yet pain is not even in the top five reasons for wanting assisted suicide in the state of Oregon. It's number six. It's listed as "pain," not "intractable pain." It's often the *fear* of pain. There are studies, Diane, that show that the more pain you have, the less interested in assisted suicide you are. I have yet to meet a patient with a late-stage terminal illness who has intractable pain.

I have lots of patients with chronic pain who aren't terminal and who have intractable pain, and who aren't happy with the approach we've had for the last thirty years of giving people opioids and fentanyl. You see what a disaster that's led to.

In terms of those who are terminal, we can use pain medication without worry, because we can escalate the dose. I rarely have to refer to pain management for terminal patients. For my late wife, pushing morphine allowed her to relax. The data show that when you give a person morphine, you don't make the person die more quickly. You allow the person to be at ease, relaxed, and they actually live longer. So, if you're doing it with the intent to help the person, that's great. And if a side effect is that they die more quickly, it's okay. You weren't trying to end their life. That wasn't the goal. The goal was to relieve their suffering. When people feel that life isn't worth living, we should give them the same love and care you gave your late husband, and live with them in the final days of life.

D: It's so interesting that you continue to use the phrase *assisted suicide,* while others who support medical aid in dying use different words.

DR. T: Words are important. All social engineering is preceded by verbal engineering. In the King's English, if you take an overdose, as a patient of mine did just a week ago, it's suicide. I'm arguing against her misguided judgment at that time. I aid the dying as they are close to death. If we're talking about death with dignity, my dad died with dignity. He was in the hospital when he passed away, surrounded by my brother and me, holding vigil.

D: I want to go back to the woman you said tried to commit suicide. You called her judgment "misguided." The issue may be: Whose judgment is it? Is it hers for herself, or is it yours as a doctor, in calling her judgment "misguided"?

DR. T: Well, I say it's misguided. And right now she would say it's misguided. But at the time, she didn't. People change their minds. As a doctor, by the way, I'm empowered. I have a power that's not present in forty-one other states. That can be very dangerous. It's an inherent conflict of interest. If we as a society want to do this, why not make it the responsibility of somebody who has some expertise in this? I had no training. Zero. In fact, one of my colleagues, who heads an oncology department in Salem, our capital, testified in public just weeks ago. He was proud of the fact that he was doing more assisted suicides in the state of Oregon than anybody else. He's a medical oncologist, for heaven's sakes. He's a talented, gifted doctor. But he's had no training in assisted suicide.

He and his anesthesiology colleagues are trying to make a cocktail that can be injected. He was testifying because the law right now says the medication has to be ingested. They're trying to change the word *ingest* to mean the medication could be injected or it could be given rectally.

D: Otherwise, everything in Oregon is going swimmingly, right? There's no slippery slope.

DR. T: The Canadians know better, Diane. They studied our law and recognized that there were people who lived for hours after the overdose with agonal breathing. They knew it was not very efficient. The Dutch know this, too. Eighty percent of the deaths in the Netherlands are done by euthanasia, direct injection. So there are all but a handful of doctors injecting people, because if you want to end people's

332

lives, and I don't, that's the efficient way to do it, as with the death penalty. You give a tranquilizer to calm the person down, then you give a barbiturate, a sedative so they go to sleep, and then you give them a muscle-paralyzing agent, so they can't breathe, their heart stops, and they're dead. Now they even want to have doctors carrying a backup kit in case that doesn't work. And they're already doing it. There have already been six thousand people across Canada who've been euthanized. As of last year, there were only five people who had done it using the Oregon method, by taking an overdose. Because it's not necessarily pretty.

I recall the case of Lovelle Svart, which was featured in *The Oregonian,* a statewide newspaper. She had cancer, and for months she kept a video log, talking about how she was going to end her life. She finally got the medication, and in the video, she holds it up. Finally, in the last scene in her life, she's having a party in her apartment. She's surrounded by friends. I have a picture of her with a friend that I often show when I'm talking about this, and you can't tell which of them is about to die. Because they're all having a good time, and she's really enjoying herself.

Thirty minutes later, she's in the bedroom. They don't make a video of this, for reasons of taste, but they have audio. She's being coached, not by a doctor, not by a nurse, but by someone who at the time was the executive director of so-called Compassion & Choices. And he's saying, "You're sure you want to do this, Lovelle?" She says, "I'd really rather go on dancing."

And he says, "You can." And she says, "No, I've already taken the anti-emetic," which keeps you from vomiting the toxic bitter medication that's going to kill her. "I'm going to go through with it." And so she does. She starts drinking it.

Her last words, or almost her last words, were "This is the most god-awful stuff I've ever tasted." Then she asks, "How am I doing?" You don't want to drink it too fast because you might vomit it. And you don't want to drink it too slowly because you might fall asleep before you take a lethal dose. He says, "You're doing fine," like this is a clinical lab experiment. He's totally dispassionate. And this is my point. Had she said that to me, I might have said something like "Lovelle, you've got a lot of life in you. Look at today, the party. You know, this is wrongheaded. I don't think this is a good idea. We can always give you more antiemetic later. Lovelle, let's think about this and do this later."

Now, this is not theoretical. One of my colleagues had a patient who had a cancer that was inoperable, a colorectal cancer. She'd gone to the surgeon, and he referred her to one of my colleagues at OHSU. She told him, "I'm not here for treatment. I'm not going to go through radiation and chemotherapy. I'm not going to have my hair fall out. I'm just here for the pills. I voted for assisted suicide Measure 16, which was the first initiative. I'm just here for the pills."

Instead of just going along with her wishes, my colleague said, "Tell me about that." He found out she had a son who was in the police academy who wasn't married. So he replied, "Don't you want to see him graduate, don't you want to see him get married?" She went home, thought about it, and the next week, she said, "You know, I think I do want the treatment." So she goes through the treatment, radiation, and chemotherapy. Her hair falls out, but it grows back. She recognizes him in a restaurant five years later and says, "Doctor, you saved my life. Had you been one of the assisted-suicide doctors, I wouldn't be here." And she's still alive, nineteen years later.

D: I know you are a devout Roman Catholic.

DR. T: Striving to be.

D: How much does your religious belief motivate your thinking?

DR. T: It's in sync with my thinking. The motto, or the slogan, for our Physicians for Compassionate Care group says that we're affirming an ethic that all human life is inherently valuable. I believe we can affirm people's worth until they die naturally. I think we can keep them comfortable. That was the whole motivation of Dame Cicely Saunders in forming hospices, to allow people to live well until they die. That's my goal in life. I want you, as a patient, to know that you don't have to worry about my motives. I'm not going to do things to you, Diane, that you don't want done. I'm not going to prolong life disproportionately. There's a time when you have to say uncle. And I'm totally open to that. But I'm going to help you live well until you die naturally. You're not going to suffer. If I can't help you, I've got colleagues who can help you. I've never had a case in which somebody couldn't get help, because we're not dealing with chronic nonterminal pain. I want people who have disabilities — whether it's speech, hearing, mobility — to realize that their life is worthwhile. Yes, my faith happens to be in sync with that. All human life is inherently valuable, I say.

D: What about the situation that Brittany Maynard found herself in? She's the young woman who moved from California to Oregon, who had a severe brain tumor that had metastasized, established residence, and lived here with her husband and mother. She was suffering from terrible problems, not only pain, but all kinds of difficulties. She tried everything. She finally said,

"I've had enough."

DR. T: She was the poster child for the assisted-suicide movement. She was a twenty-nine-year-old otherwise healthy individual who had to go through a lot of things that were not going to be curative, just like the things my wife had to go through that weren't curative. Had I been Brittany Maynard's husband or doctor, I would have done exactly what I've been sharing with you. I would have shown her her worth, her need to work on palliative care.

D: Dr. Toffler, suppose a patient with a terminal diagnosis came to you, not knowing about your belief that every life is inherently valuable, and asked you for a recommendation to a doctor who would help him or her with medical aid in dying. What would you say or do? Would you recommend another doctor?

DR. T: There's such a thing as active participation in something that is an inherent conflict of interest, and then there's passive participation. Suppose you and I were blacksmiths back in 1850, and by the grace of God and the South, we understood the evil of slavery. If somebody comes to us with their slave and asks us, "Can you fix the shackles? He ran away and damaged his shackles," we would say, because we have this insight about the inherent value of even slaves, "Sorry. I can't help you with that." He throws a rant and rage, and he's cussing at us because we won't help him. Then he says, "Okay, can you help me get to the next blacksmith? Where's the nearest one?" So, Diane, are we going to help him? If you and I believe it's misguided, are we going to compromise our integrity? Back then, we thought some people's lives were inferior to others', and we're paying for that mistake to this day. I want to treat people equally.

Diane, I don't recommend this, but you have the power to end your life. It's not rocket science. I know. I was a neurospace engineer. I'm not recommending this. I won't even go so far as to tell you the simple, everyday thing you can find at a grocery store that costs less than ten dollars and would do it. When I hear somebody having these desperate thoughts, I don't want to treat them differently because they're labeled terminal by some other doctor who thinks they're terminal.

D: Now that Maine's Death with Dignity Act has gone into effect, do you think we're on a path to fifty states being willing to accept it?

DR. T: No, I don't. There are actually at least ten states that have strengthened their laws against assisted suicide. Barring the Supreme Court stepping in, as they did in Canada, I do not see all states embracing this. Maine Governor Janet Mills said, "I hope this isn't used much." Well, what can she possibly be thinking? It's expanded in Oregon. There are well over 1,500 cases there, over 6,600 cases in Canada. It's gone up threefold in the last fourteen years in the Netherlands. She's not looking at facts.

If it's medical aid while dying, I'm in agreement with it. If it's death with dignity, I'm in agreement with it. But we're talking about empowering doctors to give massive doses or injections, as some of my colleagues want to do here in Oregon. They're already doing it in Canada, the Netherlands, and Belgium, and it's the identical treatment we give to serial killers on death row. Whether you believe in the death penalty or not, that's not the point. The point is, if it's supposedly cruel and unusual punishment, as some people say about the death penalty, how is it compassionate care when it's a totally innocent person? You have to tie yourself into a pretzel to justify this. It's exactly the same series of drugs.

D: What would a good death be for you?

DR. T: Surrounded by family, loved ones, supporting me with the amount of intervention and care that I desire. I *used* to think I would like to die on a racquetball court, and just have a quick, easy death.

ALLAN CHRISTOPHER CARMICHAEL

RETIRED ASSOCIATE DIRECTOR OF
COLLECTIONS AND HORTICULTURE AT THE
UC BOTANICAL GARDEN
WIDOWER OF TERRY STEIN

&

DR. STEPHANIE MARQUET

TERRY STEIN'S PALLIATIVE CARE
PHYSICIAN

As I walk up to the front door of Chris Carmichael's home, it is clear that a gifted gardener has designed the entrance. There is a lovely "natural" garden, with flowers, ferns, and plantings one doesn't ordinarily see on the East Coast. The doorway is beautifully surrounded by greenery and seems to welcome passersby to take a closer look. Later, we view the back garden, which has its own rare and breathtaking beauty.

Chris is the designer, and the surviving spouse of Terry Sheldon Stein, who died six months before this interview took place. Chris is tall and slender, with a bearded and mustachioed face.

I ask how he and Terry first met.

CHRIS: We met in East Lansing, Michigan, where he was an associate professor of psychiatry and I was a master's student, but we were only eight years apart in age. Terry was on the faculty of the medical school, a psychotherapist, was very involved in gay and lesbian cultural politics for many years, working on the pathological diagnosis of homosexuality, and determined to remove the last vestiges of that classification.

We had a very rich thirty-eight-year relationship together. He, or we, had a son, Martin, by a previous marriage. I met Martin when he was eight years old, and together, we jointly raised him with his mother and her husband. And that was a very big part of Terry's identity, being a dad, as well as a grandfather, now that Martin has four children.

Terry took an early retirement and we moved to the Bay Area because of its cultural politics, but also because Terry was very involved in Zen Buddhism and very attracted to the Zen communities here.

DIANE: What were the first indications

that Terry was not well?

C: In the summer of 2015, Terry was diagnosed with mild cognitive impairment.

D: How did that manifest itself?

C: Well, Terry was a psychiatrist, and a certified neurologist, too. And there was a period of time when he kept asking questions over and over again. Or, he would ask a question and lose his train of thought. And we both thought, Well, this is odd, but maybe we should have it looked into. We were sort of cavalier about it. But the tests came back showing a clear diagnosis of low-level mild cognitive impairment. And one of the big challenges with that was that Terry's mother died of dementia, and he was very determined not to slide into dementia. But when it comes to the end-of-life option, dementia or psychological impairment prohibits one from accessing it. And he was very upset about that. One of his biggest fears was descending into dementia without having the option of choosing not to.

D: So then, he was diagnosed with another condition?

C: Right. A year later, almost to the day

of the first diagnosis, he was diagnosed with advanced bladder cancer, and it had metastasized widely, which had not been immediately apparent when he started treatment. I would never use the term *relief,* and yet it's hard not to. He was relieved that he would have a medically appropriate diagnosis if he needed, so that he would not suffer through either of his illnesses.

D: I understand you and he had already talked about medical aid in dying and that he'd had a friend who had died, and he was determined that he would not die in the same way?

C: Right. That's true. He was very, very clear about the importance of having agency in making his end-of-life choices. He had several friends who had looked at the option, including Lillian Rubin, the author and psycho-therapist. She was extremely clear about her end-of-life wishes, and Terry was one of her major supports along the way. He learned a lot about the process and became committed to sup-porting Lillian in her choices. He also developed an interest in seeing the limitations decrease so that people with a broader range of afflictions could access the end-of-life treatment.

D: When did Terry contact Compassion & Choices?

C: Early on. After his diagnosis of mild cognitive impairment, and after his diagnosis of bladder cancer. He had very helpful conversations with the folks at Compassion & Choices, but the only option they were really offering or encouraging was to withhold liquid and forgo food. He didn't find that personally helpful.

D: Dr. Marquet, tell me about the first interaction you had with Terry.

DR. MARQUET: I came here to the home to meet Terry and his family, Chris, and whoever else had wanted to be present would have been welcomed. I'd like to address the amount of pre-work that happens before a physician engages with a patient about medical aid in dying. Chris has mentioned mild cognitive impairment, and we all know that the lack of capacity excludes a person from medical aid in dying. It's a very important point to consider and, as a physician, to absorb. I had to meet Terry to really know the situation and to know his heart. And to know his cognitive status, though it was clear from the record that Terry absolutely had the full capacity to understand his medical condition, to be driving the boat of his care, to weigh treatment options, and to understand their consequences. He was very articulate with his cancer physician and had multiple visits with his palliative-care team.

Before I met Terry, I had the privilege of learning about him from his medical record, which was very in-depth, because he was a very intellectual man who did not take anything for granted. I assume, given his mild cognitive impairment, that he did well with laying out facts concretely. You could see from the way clinicians were documenting conversations with him that he was relying on concrete facts as guideposts. So I was not surprised, when I met Terry in person, that we had a very rich and long conversation about his journey with his sudden illness. When patients are talking about what it's like to live with their terminal diagnosis, I like their being able to walk me through that journey with them. Terry was really hoping that the treatments would provide a medical cure. He had gotten multiple opinions to determine the best surgery, and he did go through extensive surgery. But several months after his surgery, his cancer had metastasized to the liver.

C: And to the bone.

DR. M: His bones. That was very painful. I remember some of these details because Terry was giving me the gift of walking me through what it was like for him to hope for more time. Cancer is a scary diagnosis, but the doctors are telling him that, with treatment, he can have more time, and he wanted more time. But then it became clear that his cancer was not curable, and his treatment options were very limited. A high treatment burden to a low chance of providing more quality time. Often, as I work with people interested in medical aid in dying, there is some guiding sense of self, and Terry absolutely had that. He was able to articulate to me so well why he didn't like the phrase *being in charge,* because as a Buddhist, he didn't think being in charge was important; it was more being open to the reality of what was happening to him. In making the choice from the options available to him, there was one that resonated. It was medical aid in dying.

D: And, Chris, to what extent did you and Terry deliberate about that choice?

C: It was apparent that it was very important to him to have that alternative. I would say we talked about it a lot, but he was so clear and articulate about his wishes, and the palliative-care team supported him. They had seldom dealt with someone so articulate and straightforward about what they wanted and could talk about their feelings, too, not just the nuts and bolts.

D: Dr. Marquet, what kind of training did you have to be involved with medical aid in dying?

DR. M: This work is new. We're only two years in. When I met Terry, I had one year of experience with medical aid in dying. Overall, I've had twenty years of experience, and working with the dying requires a special skill set. I worked ten years as a hospitalist, dealing with acute medical crises, and another ten years in palliative medicine and hospice care. Both have influenced me and given me confidence. Doing the work well has also required experiential learning. When I met Terry, I was working for Kaiser, and Kaiser has done a great job at providing education to the practitioners who opt to participate. Just as patients have a choice to take advantage of medical aid in dying, so does each person on the medical side. Kaiser as an organization opted to participate and offer medical aid in dying, but then it was up to the physicians, the nurses, the hospice groups, to say whether they wanted to know more and potentially work with patients one-on-one.

I was one of the people early on who received training about both the law and Kaiser policy, some talking points, the required elements, as well as access to an end-of-life-options patient coordinator, who is considered Kaiser's expert in medical aid in dying.

As a physician, I find it very interesting that in most encounters with patients, we decide together what's best for them, and in working within the context of medical aid in dying, there is a third party — the law, in a sense, the state. And I can speak for the whole team that worked with Terry, we wanted to be absolutely compliant with the law, but it makes things a little jerkier — at one point, I had to ask Chris to leave, because there's a requirement in the law to speak privately one-on-one.

D: Even though Terry and Chris were married?

DR. M: Absolutely. It's required in the law that there be a private moment, one-on-one, to confirm that this is indeed Terry's own wish. I used that time to ask if there was anything he'd like to share with me without the presence of his family, not only whether it was really his choice, but about hopes and fears that he didn't feel comfortable sharing with his family.

D: How many patients have you seen through the entire process?

DR. M: I've worked with probably fifteen patients now. I've attended one death by medical aid in dying, but as one of the physician leads, I've worked with more than that as a support to my colleagues, and as an educator to my colleagues as well.

D: Chris, was Dr. Marquet with you and Terry on the last day of Terry's life?

C: At that point, Dr. Marquet had stepped back. We had worked together to obtain the medication and to understand its use just a few days before his actual death. And Terry's last day was one of the hardest things in this whole process. But one of the most satisfying things is that you know when you're going to die. You make the decision about when that seems right in the context of your family, your friends, and your loved ones. Terry was very intent on not suffering, and also not making those around him suffer in the process.

D: Who was here with you on the day Terry died?

C: There was a whole support team to be with both of us. Terry's son, Martin Stein, was here and held Terry's hand until the end. And three very good friends, one of whom is an internist, one of whom is a retired hospice nurse, and the third person, who was his closest friend. He had the people who meant the most with him. The day of Terry's death is hard for me to look back on. He never wavered in terms of knowing what he wanted, and I shared his opinions about the end-of-life option. I support it fully, and yet it didn't make it any easier, the actual death. I'd ask how he was feeling, and he said he was okay but that he couldn't talk much about what was going to happen because he was afraid he'd lose his nerve. I never saw him waver, so his answer was a bit startling. And he didn't. He didn't lose his nerve.

THE HONORABLE SELWA "LUCKY" ROOSEVELT

CHIEF OF PROTOCOL IN THE REAGAN ADMINISTRATION

Selwa "Lucky" Roosevelt was born in Tennessee, the daughter of Lebanese Druze immigrants. She spent her youth there, went to Vassar College, and just before graduating, met Archibald "Archie" B. Roosevelt, Jr. They met on a Saturday, and he asked her to marry him on Sunday. They were married three months later. They spent their first years together overseas, then returned to Washington, where they lived for four years. Various government assignments took them overseas again, but they finally settled in Washington, D.C. They were married for forty years, until he died in 1979. Lucky Roosevelt and I live in the same condominium and have become good friends. This interview took place in her beautiful and comfortable apartment, where there are many photographs of her and her adored husband. When we spoke, Lucky was about to celebrate her ninetieth birthday.

DIANE: Lucky, I understand your mother lived in this very building prior to your moving here.

LUCKY: That's correct. She came from Tennessee to be with me, and my sister was in New York. The two of us looked after her, but then in her last years, she couldn't stay in the apartment. We moved her to an assisted living facility, and then when she developed dementia, we had to move her to another section of the facility, where she died.

D: I know that you testified before the District of Columbia Council when they were considering the medical-aid-in-dying measure. Was the death of your mother, and how she died, a motivating factor in the development of your own thinking?

L: Absolutely. It was, for me, such a tragedy and such a lack of dignity. This is a woman who had done so much in her life and was such a loving and productive person. She died at ninety-eight, but she had these terrible four or five years before she died. And this is what really devastated me, to see this incredibly productive, wonderful woman disintegrate. It made me so anxious to do anything I could to help

355

other people avoid going through what I did with my mother. I have been very conscious of the importance of dying with dignity ever since.

D: Did you and your husband ever talk about this?

L: Well, yes, we did. I was quite young when he died, but I was spared so much. He died of a heart attack in his sleep. I didn't even know it was happening. And the next morning when I woke up, he was gone. Of course, it was devastating, that sense of loss was enormous, but I always think what good fortune for him that he had a painless death. It was God's gift.

D: Can you summarize for me what you said to the D.C. Council?

L: Basically, how important I thought it was for people to die in — I keep using the word *dignity,* which is so important to me and to everyone else, I guess — to not die in an indescribably awful way, which is what happens when people are not allowed to die when they want to die. My mother told me before she became completely demented, she said, "It's time for me to go." She knew that it was time for her to go, and she asked me if I could help her. And I knew I couldn't because I knew the law. And I knew she wouldn't want me to end up in jail. I told her that, and she was very upset with me because she felt that I should help her go. But I didn't know how to. I'm so grateful that now there's a possibility of helping others. I was really disappointed that every single one of the doctors who testified was against passage of the law. We have every right to make our own decisions. Why should anyone else make those decisions for us?

D: What about helping yourself?

L: Well, I don't know what's going to happen to me yet, but I plan to make it as — I hope I can make it as swift and meaningful as possible. I want death not to be a horror story for me. I've been blessed with good health, and I don't know how it'll end, but I'm hoping that by the time I'm ready to go, the laws will be changed all over the country and people won't have to fly to Switzerland and other places to be able to have a death that one could live with.

It's so hard to talk about it, really. But it's essential that this country be awakened to the importance of this. I think it's wonderful what you're doing, Diane. I really admire you for that. I think this is the way to go. The group Compassion & Choices has the right attitude and the right cause. I believe in it.

D: Lucky, I have my own ideas of what would be a good death. I wonder what yours are.

L: A heart attack would be my preferred way of going. But that's not likely. I think I would want to be able, at the point of death or possibly when it was not so far off, I would like to be able to say to my doctor and to my family and everybody who cared, that it's time for me to go. I would like to have that choice, and I would like to be able to take a medication myself, some pill or whatever is the right thing to do, and I would like to die that way. I feel that very, very strongly.

D: Have you actually talked with your doctor about what you'd like?

L: He's not very receptive. I'm going to have to work on him. I have told him that there's a list of things: no resuscitation, no this, no that. I don't want any emergency measures they do in the hospital. I refuse to go to a hospital that doesn't allow you to die without all those machines. I told my doctor that. He has to take me to a specific hospital.

D: Did he understand that?

L: He would be willing to put me in the hospital that doesn't have to have those terrible things that they do to people to keep them alive when they're half dead. I don't want any of that. I would prefer to die in my own home, in my own bed, if that were possible. I'm hoping I'll have nurses and people to look after me if I'm sick. You never know. It's so hard to plan for. You don't know where you might be, what might be your illness that would be the cause of death. The worst thing is dementia, which Mother had. But she knew that it was time, and she knew things weren't going very well in her mental state. I'm hoping that I would know.

D: I feel the same way. As a matter of fact, I have told my children and my grandchildren that what I would like to have is a gathering in my apartment and for everyone to be cheerful and loving. And toasting each other, and then I would quietly go off to my bedroom with my husband and children and grandchildren and say goodbye.

L: That would be the ideal way for me. You described it perfectly. That couldn't be better. And I think it's so cruel of the legislators and the people who oppose this. They don't understand.

D: What is it you think they don't understand?

L: They don't understand how important it is in your own soul, your own feeling, that you want to go, the way God intended you to go. I mean if you're religious, and I'm not particularly, but if you are religious, you must believe that God didn't intend you to suffer needlessly, and that you should go when the right time comes. Now, as you know, various legislators are motivated by all kinds of religious beliefs and other things. They don't see the tragedy and the incredible pain associated with not letting people go when they are ready.

D: Tell me how you felt when you learned that the law in D.C. had finally passed.

L: I was thrilled. I was so pleased that I

went down and testified. I told them how I felt and how important I thought it was. And I thought it was just wonderful that our legislature had the guts to do what is not right now the most popular thing to do. So many states haven't got the courage so far. But I think it's going to happen.

D: Why do you think that?

L: Because it's the logical and the right thing to do. Sooner or later, some of these legislators, the ones who are so adamantly opposed, are going to have to face it themselves, and they're going to find out how important it is to be able to die with dignity.

D: If you were terminally ill, and if you realized in advance that you were not going to get better, do you feel you would have your doctor's support for how you want to go?

L: You've asked me a tough question because I'm not absolutely sure, but as I've said, I'm going to work on my doctors and make them more and more receptive to the idea.

D: It seems to me that as a former chief of protocol of the United States, you would have the right words to do that.

L: Well, I've talked with my doctor about

it and I think he just isn't . . . I think so many doctors need to be educated in this. It isn't part of their medical training. They think their mission, in the days of approaching death, is to keep you alive no matter what. It's time for them to realize that that's not what is best for their patients. Even twenty years ago, people died around eighty. Now it's amazing how many people live to their nineties. It's important for doctors to rethink what they were taught in medical school, because things have changed.

D: Looking at you, Lucky, no one would ever guess how close you are to being ninety years old.

L: I know. I'm healthy. I mean, I'm so lucky.

D: Where did the nickname Lucky come from?

L: I got it in college, because I was a very good bridge player. And they all didn't attribute it to my ability to play bridge; they attributed it to my lucky cards. Everybody called me Lucky, even my mother, finally. It's a name I love because I really feel that I'm lucky. And I just hope that it'll extend to the day I'm facing death.

BENJAMIN ZIDE

SOPHOMORE, DARTMOUTH COLLEGE, GRANDSON OF DIANE REHM

Benjamin Zide is my grandson. At the time this conversation was recorded, Ben was eighteen years old. He'd come to Washington to spend a part of his spring vacation with me, which totally delighted and flattered me. How many men of Ben's age want to spend time with their aging grandmothers? But from the time he was a toddler, we have had a wonderful and loving relationship. His mother (my daughter, Jennifer) likes to tell the story that when my late husband and I would visit their family in Boston, Ben would weep uncontrollably when it was time for us to leave. At the time of this recording, Ben was a senior at Concord Academy. He is now an undergraduate at Dartmouth. Before we had this conversation, I had asked his mother's permission, which she granted.

DIANE: Ben, I want to talk with you about something. Do you have your iPhone with you?

BEN: Yeah.

D: Ben, I'd like you to record our conversation on your iPhone, so you have it, your mother has it, your father has it, and your uncle Dave (my son), Aunt Nancy, and my husband, John Hagedorn, have it, okay? I want everybody to know exactly how I feel about what I'd like at the end of life.

B: And you want me to record it?

D: Please. You can start recording now. A few months ago, I came across a perfect paragraph that Anne Morrow Lindbergh had left behind, and her daughter Reeve Lindbergh found after her mother died. It just encapsulated so beautifully what I want for myself. And, Ben, after I read this, if you have questions, we can talk about it. Is that okay with you?

B: Sounds good to me.

D: Okay. She wrote, "To my family, my physician, and my hospital: If there is no reasonable expectation of my recovery from mental or physical disability, I request I be allowed to die and not be kept alive by artificial means and heroic measures. I ask that medication be mercifully administered to me for terminal suffering, even if it hastens the moment of my death. I hope that you who care for me will feel morally bound to act in accordance with this urgent request."

So that's what Anne Morrow Lindbergh wrote. And when I read it, I thought, Wow, that's exactly how I feel. If, for example, I develop Alzheimer's disease, and know that I have Alzheimer's, or you begin to notice, I want you to tell me, "DeeDee, you're failing, you're losing it a little bit, I can see that." I want you to tell me that. I want everybody in our family to tell me that. I want to know when I am failing, so that when I reach a point where I know I'm going straight downhill, I want to go peacefully. If I am physically disabled so that I can no longer care for myself, I can no longer feed myself, I can no longer bathe myself or take care of myself in any way, I don't want to be in a nursing home, I want to die peacefully and quietly.

Now, I'm going to arrange for that myself, but what I would really like is for the whole family to be here on that last day of my life, so I can be with all of you, together. We will laugh, we will enjoy each other's company, we will be with each other in happiness, and then I will go into my bedroom and into my own bed and I will pass away. And that will be a very happy moment for me if it can happen that way. And of course I will want John, my husband, to be here as well. He will want to be with me. So are you okay with that?

B: I'm okay with that.

D: Do you have any questions you want to ask me?

B: Yeah. If you are not physically capable of ending your own life, whose responsibility would it be?

D: By then, my darling, I figure you will be sufficiently trained as a medical expert to know when my end is coming close. And if I have not been able to take care of it myself, I will hope that one of you will be able to help me with that. I so believe in medical aid in dying and my right to choose the time and place of my death that that's how I'd like it to be. And I hope that if there is any disagreement among any of you that my wishes will prevail and that one of you will be able to help me.

B: And if you're physically still capable, but mentally incapable — how are we to determine when your mental incapability is advanced to the degree that you no longer wish to continue?

D: I think that there will have to be a discussion between you and me, perhaps your mother and me, your uncle Dave and John and me. We will know when the time comes, when it's so close that I can no longer be of use to myself, to you, to society. We will know when that end comes. And I am asking for love and cooperation and careful judgment on everybody's part.

B: Okay.

D: Ben, I realize everything I'm saying is putting a great deal of responsibility on you because you're here with me as we film this conversation. And filming it not only for me, but for posterity. I'm eighty-one years old now. Who knows how long I might have. I have no idea. I realize that talking to you this way, when you're eighteen years old, is putting a lot on your shoulders. How does all this make you feel?

B: It makes my heart beat a lot faster than I wish it did. I think of losing Bee

367

[his grandfather, John Rehm], who was my greatest mentor and person I looked up to in life. Watching him go physically but not mentally was something I never wish to see again. And then losing my other grandmother to Alzheimer's is something I wish I never have to see again. So I plan on making sure that however you would like to end is what I support completely. I know both Bee and my grandmother would never have wished to see themselves in the state they were in at the end. And if you don't want to either, I completely understand. Even though this is an uncomfortable conversation right now, it's an important one.

D: You're right, and I appreciate your putting it that way. Ben, I want your mother and father and Uncle Dave and Aunt Nancy and John all to have this on video. And you mustn't think of this as sad, because I keep thinking, This is all part of life. Your grandfather said, "I'm looking forward to the next journey." I'm convinced there *is* a next journey, and I want you to think of it in that way as well.

ACKNOWLEDGMENTS

When I first met Bob Gottlieb in 1996, I had no idea he would be in my life and in my head for the next two decades. From the beginning, he has educated and helped me, not only as a writer but as a guide through this complicated journey called living. I will be ever thankful to have had the good fortune to have him as my editor as well as my friend.

Sonny Mehta, the head of Knopf, took a chance on me all those years ago, and is once again putting his strength and support behind this book. Since the very early days of my radio career, Paul Bogaards and I have worked together happily and successfully. He has been and continues to be a champion of my work as both broadcaster and writer.

Special thanks to Marc Jaffee, who helped in every way, including editorially.

Also at Knopf, my thanks to Lydia

Buechler, Susan Brown, Peggy Samedi, Betty Lew, Kelly Blair, and Emily Murphy.

For Rebecca Kaufman and Alison Brody, I offer gratitude for their taking on so much responsibility for the creation and formation of our podcast, *On My Mind.* And to JJ Yore, the best manager at WAMU I've ever had.

Finally, Joe Fab and Diane Naughton came to me with the idea of a documentary on the right to die two years ago, and generously allowed me to use many of the transcripts from that documentary to create this book; and Dave Goulding, whose talent as a man behind the camera managed to make me look good.

ABOUT THE AUTHOR

Diane Rehm hosted *The Diane Rehm Show,* distributed by NPR, from 1979 to 2016, when it had a listening audience of two-and-a-half million. She now hosts a podcast for WAMU-NPR, *On My Mind.* She lives in Washington, D.C.